Please *Educate Yourself*

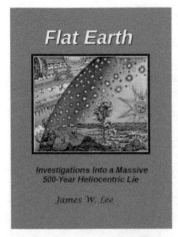

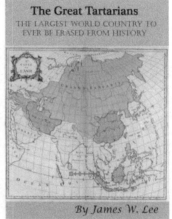

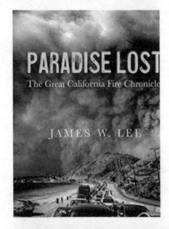

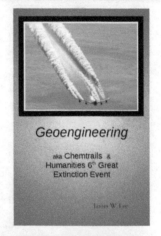

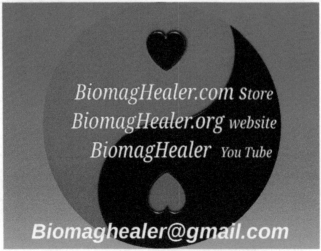

Dedications

There are few Pioneers recognized in the healing arts today towards our common destiny of Spiritual Science healing for all.

The first modern day hero of non-invasive Subtly Energetic Vibrational Healing is Dr. Randolph Stone (1890-1981), who Bioneered "Polarity Therapy" to adjust and adapt the body energetically using opposing positive and negative magnetic energies to achieve optimal healing and wellness. Dr. Stone ended up moving to India to live in an Ashram after being ridiculed and abused by the western medicine community for his work in Biomag Healing.

A couple decades later Dr. Goiz (1941-2021), from Mexico, introduced Biomagnetic Polarity Therapy (BPT) and developed, and greatly furthered the art of subtle energy healing and began teaching others how to use magnets to heal as well as develop a systematic BiomagHealing protocol. He greatly advanced our knowledge of how to heal using magnets and set about teaching others what he had learned. His first soul he helped was a man suffering from AIDS, or in reality the Burroughs Welcome Inc. AZT drug that gave him the AIDS, to fully recover.

From student to teacher to professor and cutting-edge leader of Biomagnetic Healing comes Dr. Luis Garcia. Dr. Garcia has taken Dr. Goiz's work and expanded it exponentially so that it is now possible, given scalability, to achieve his stated goal of "healing the world" through Biomagnetic Healing protocols and methodologies applied energetically. For two decades, Dr. Goiz initial findings on healing with magnets, were only taught in Spanish for years and years. Dr. Garcia not only attended over 20 of Dr. Goiz's workshops but critically translated Dr. Goiz's work into English as well as put together the Greatest Healing Medical Book ever written called the "Biomag Practitioner's Guide Handbook" which can be purchased on his website at usbiomag.com. Additionally, Dr. Garcia discovered hundreds and hundreds of additional pairs of biomagnetic placements of diseases, symptoms and emotional issues adding to what Dr. Goiz found as well. Dr. Garcia is also is currently and graciously teaching hundreds of lay people, like you and me, how to use Biomag Healing skills in his intensive workshops, that anyone can learn and apply. He also continues to upgrade and add more placements of terrain and vaccine induced diseases and illness' as well as placements for over 130 emotional issues.

Lastly, I wish to dedicate my profound gratitude to the Source, Creator, God, et al. for allowing me, and all who wish to learn this amazing methodology access to this profound healing protocol. And to the angels that assist me in healing namely angelic healers Arch-Angel Michael and Green Tara. I could not, and would not, be able achieve the healing success I have to date, without their loving help and guidance. For that I am so appreciative and grateful.

"May every impulse of life flowing through us fortify the relationship between ourselves and our bodies. May we cherish our precious bodies through thought, speech, feeling and action. May the immeasurable love of the Creator, and the Absolute pure, truth of Source radiate through every particle of our amazing physical forms. May this love, truth and purity, which we are, guide our choices and decisions about self-care. May it be so."
— Dorothy Rowe

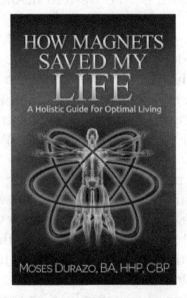

If man but understood magnetism in true,
he would seize the universe by the tail
—Nikola Tesla

A BiomagHealers Guide
To Self-Healing With Magnets

"The desire that guides me in all I do is the desire to harness the forces of nature to the service of mankind."
– Nikola Tesla

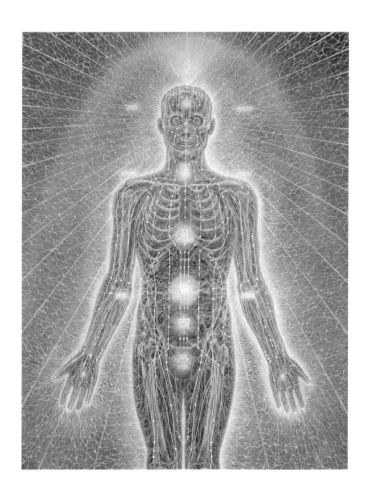

James W. Lee
6.27.21

Table of Contents

Preface   ix
> What If?

Introduction: Born2 Self-Heal   1
> Book Layout. Intention and Focus. End of All Suffering is Near and
> Here. My path to BiomagHealing.

1) What is Biomagentism?   11
> Definitions of Health. 10 Golden Rules of Biomagnetism. Effects of
> Biomagnetism on the Human Body. How Biomagnetism Works. Magnet
> Polarities. Biomagnetic Scanning.

2) Let's Heal the World   23
> What Can Biomagnetism Heal?

3) Let's Heal the World ~ Applying Biomagnetic Healing Protocols   27
> Methods of Muscle Testing. Session Work ~ Let's Begin to Heal. Remote
> Healing at a Distance

4) Principles of Biomagnetic Healing with Magnets   37
> What are Magnets. Types of Rare Earth Magnets. Magnets in Everyday
> Life. Remote Healing at a Distance with Magnets. Subtle Vibrational
> Healing Energy. Remote Viewing. Next Level of Biomag Healing ~
> Spiritual Cleansing.

5) The Deliberate Suppression in History of Biomag Healing   61
> Subtle Vibrational Energy. Chinese Book of Medicine 3000 b.c. Ka, Chi,
> Prana, Jesus Heals, The Flexner Report of 1910. Paracelsus. Franz Anton
> Mr. Rudolph Steiner & Mr. Nikola Tesla. Dr. Randolph Stone, Dr. Goiz
> & Dr. Luis Garcia

6) Biomag Agriculture ~ Super Grow More*Stronger*Faster   79
> Benefits of the application of irrigation with Magnetic treatments in
> agriculture. Magnetite. Structured Water. Magnetized Garden Beds

7) Complimentary Healing Resources   89
> Nutrition. Supplements. Vitamins. Meditation. Creams. Lotions. Potions. Detox Food and much more. Healing powers of Medical Marijuana. Heavy Metal Detox Foods.

8) Covidiocracy and the Really, Really Big Agenda of the NWO   131
> Drugged and Vaxxed to Death. Georgia Guidestones. The Really, Really Big Agenda. Magnetorecptors. All Chipped. Head in the Clouds.

Conclusion   147
> Only the Beginning, No, Not Just a Start.

Applied Biomagnetics Workbook

Appendix I   **The Question Tree**   149

Appendix II   **Scan Charts and Session Protocols**   159

Appendix III   **Testimonials**   223

Appendix IV   **Setting Up Your Business as a Biomag Healer**   229

Appendix VI   **Biomag Healer Goods and Services**   231

Bibliography   235

About the Author   237

Preface

What If ?!?
We All Can Learn to Heal
One Another and the World

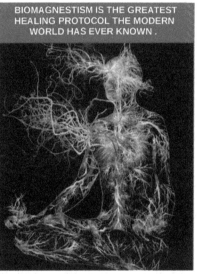

BIOMAGNESTISM IS THE GREATEST HEALING PROTOCOL THE MODERN WORLD HAS EVER KNOWN .

What if there was the Greatest Healing Protocol the world has ever known since the first book on modern medicine came out in China in 3,000 B.C., that very few are even aware of today?

What if this element we all can attain and harness, is free and abundant everywhere, to anyone, at any time, in abundance?

What if this is a non-invasive subtle energy healing protocol was proven to have been dismissed as 'quackery' in 1910 and hidden from the Western World for over 100 years and is now being reborn again for all to learn and heal one another without hospitals of doctors needed?

What if this amazing healing protocol crosses all countries, languages and race barriers?

What if anyone and everyone, at any age, can learn this most amazing healing protocol?

What if all one needed was a pair of rare earth N52 Neodymium magnets and some knowledge of where to place the magnets to remedy most any conditions and issues, whether it be physical, mental, emotional and/or Spiritual?

What if we all could heal the world together, individual by individual, and even in groups, using this ancient healing protocol?

What if Western Medicine re-learned Biomag Healing, and all doctors and healing souls would learn this most amazing healing protocol whereby hospitals closed, and the 3rd leading cause of death is greatly reduced and/or eliminated entirely?

What if we no longer needed pills, poisoned chemotherapy or poisoned radiation to rid the body of radiation and toxic poisons as well as No more huge medical bills ?

What if you no longer needed medical insurance and the medical mafia went "away" because they became obsolete?

What if this Self-Healing Protocol would eliminate the need for most surgeries, psychiatrists and therapists as well as not need the drug pushers of Big p**HARM**a?

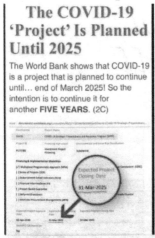

The COVID-19 'Project' Is Planned Until 2025

The World Bank shows that COVID-19 is a project that is planned to continue until... end of March 2025! So the intention is to continue it for another **FIVE YEARS**. (2C)

What if we were able to scan and detect newly lab created artificial devices implanted in our bodies and destroy or mitigate their effectiveness?

What if we could reverse the ill effects of the Covid Vaccine and over 300 GMO vaccines in the pipeline with follow up booster shots intended to be implemented through 2025?

What if this healing energy protocol enabled you to connect to the Aether, and Akashic record to access vital information to help heal each other in very profound ways in solid proof of The Interconnectedness of All to the Infinite and to each other?

What if we could heal one another remotely, at a distance, without even knowing, or meeting the person, or animal, we are intentionally focusing on to help them with their issues and ailments based on our intention and our Biomag placements???

What if we can all be taught 'to fish' and thereby heal ourselves and others for time eternal?

What if our children could learn this protocol to heal one another and themselves as well as maintain optimum health?

AND, If everyone learned to muscle test alone, we would achieve World Peace because each of us could ask the Universe any question and get honest real time answers.

Is this person telling the truth or lie? Should I do this or this? Am I in danger if I do this? etc. and get the TRUTH! No one could ever lie to us again without our knowing it and all of us would be able to each heal another, even at distance.

Think about the Potential If We All Can Learn

Let's Heal the World

*****

Introduction

Born2 Self-Heal

Allergies * Anemia * Asthma * Sinusitis * Lyme disease * Acne * Psoriasis * Migraines • HIV • Aids • Arrhythmia • Diabetes • Flu • Chronic Fatigue • Herpes • Fibromyalgia • Alzheimer's • Carpul Tunnel • Chronic Pain • Sciatica • Gastritis • Reflux • Ulcerative colitis • Crohn's disease • Cancer • Back Pain • Arthritis • Rheumatism • Varicose Veins • Poor Circulation • Digestive Disorders • Pulmonary Disorders • Skin Disorders • Fungus • Parasites • PMS • Menopause and PMS Symptoms • Glandular Dysfunctions • Adrenal Fatigue • Stress • Heartburn • Parkinson's • High Cholesterol • Impotency • Hepatitis • Sexual disorders • Infertility • Low Libido • Meningitis • Tendonitis • Tennis Elbow • pH Unbalance • Ulcers • Depression • Anxiety • Emotional Issues • Autism • Attention Deficit Disorder • Energetic Unbalances • and many others....

Just a few of the many, many issues BiomagHealing addresses

Book Layout and Format

This book is designed to be educational as well as how to begin to apply Biomag-Healing principles and protocols and how we all can use the power of magnetism to optimize health.

My hope is that this will begin a whole new and wonderful healing chapter in you and your families lives since everyone and anyone can learn this amazing healing with magnets. The book begins with explaining the history and nuts n' bolts of Biomag healing as well as how magnets work and why. This is followed by my historical narrative of the origins and resurrection now of Biomagetic Healing as well as current proof of how and why biomagnetism is effective and successful in its applications.

The Appendixes sections are intended to be for your session work to help guide you in scanning and placements as well as how to conduct a healing session and what questions to ask to get profound lasting results.

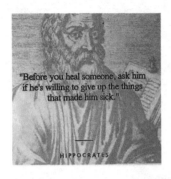

"Before you heal someone, ask him if he's willing to give up the things that made him sick."

HIPPOCRATES

Caution: Not everyone is ready to benefit from BiomagHealing. Unless the soul wishes to change the behaviors that caused the illness', intake of toxic foods, emotional disruptions and lifestyles that brought on the issues and ailments in the first place, then the BiomagHealer will only effect temporary change in many cases. It is critical that the soul you are assisting to facilitate their healing is asked, "Do you wish to do what is necessary to self-heal"? If you get a no, do not do placements until you can get an affirmative that it is okay to help and assist.

This book is intended to be an entrée level guide to help you get started and learn how to become effective and efficient at healing yourself and others, even at a distance. You will learn how to muscle scan, apply magnets to individuals for their unique needs and issues as well as to develop your own unique healing protocols that can, and should, be applied with most other forms of homeopathy. If we all can learn this incredible protocol, and heal ourselves and loved ones, we will take down the machine once and for all. Period!

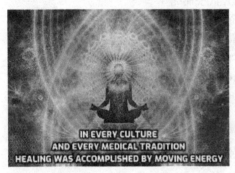

IN EVERY CULTURE AND EVERY MEDICAL TRADITION HEALING WAS ACCOMPLISHED BY MOVING ENERGY

This healing protocol is only now being reconstituted in modern day healing and has been used by the Ancient Ones, by the first modern medicine healers of China, the Vedics of India, the pyramidic creating Egyptians and even Jesus Christ in his last act of compassion to his Apostles before being crucified!

Learning to muscle test is critical or the use of dowsing, and/or hands on healing also works well to determine what issues and symptoms need to be addressed and where to put on the magnet pairs. We are just in the embryonic stages of Biomag Healing which means there is much to learn and much to explore about what is possible to help and to heal ourselves, our loved ones and possibly, entire group healing set with intention.

Intentions and Focus

Etymology: intention (n.) late 14c., entencioun, "purpose, design, aim or object; will, wish, desire, that which is intended, from Latin intentionem (nominative intentio) "a stretching out, straining, exertion, effort; attention," noun of action from intendere "to turn one's attention," literally "to stretch out" (see intend). Also in Middle English "emotion, feelings; heart, mind, mental faculties, understanding."

One of the most basic of BiomagHealing protocols is to how you use your intentions and if you have a clear mind and body in order to assist and facilitate healing of the souls you are working with.

With your intention you can set the magnets to affect remedy in general or in very specific areas of the mind and body down to the cellular level. Focus is critical as well so that your mind is clear and your body a tool, a vehicle, for the Spirit beings to help guide and assist you through the healing process using magnets. Your intentions are what directs the subtle energy where it needs to go. Are you intending to do a general placement, or is there a vein, artery, nerve, ligament, bone, etc. that needs to be targeted with magnetic energy? If you get a "yes" from muscle scanning, then you simply set your intention as to where the magnetic energy is specifically targeted to go. The more focused your intention, the more effective the results.

Also, the more you learn about the anatomy of the body, the more effective your intentions will be for optimal healing and well being. Concluding a session you can also set your intention to command the body to heal, spoken orally or silently.

You will also want to ensure that you stay connected to the soul you are facilitating their own healing. If you break from focusing, simply ask to be reconnected to the soul by muscle testing.

End of All Suffering is Near and Here

Finally, the end of Suffering is the last of the Tibetan 4 noble truths and that is EXACTLY what Biomagnetism has the potential to do for all worldwide, including pets, flora and fauna…and **The End of Suffering for All**. We now have the answers to optimal healing and well-being once more.

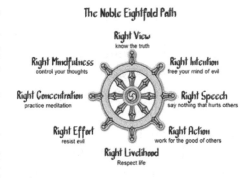

According to Vedic traditions, the oldest known writings of man, suffering is the root cause of all illness

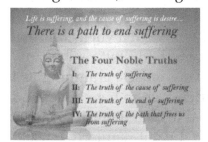

and dis-eases. Ending suffering ends the cyclic karma accumulated once and for all.

Just as the darkness of the World Elite using a fake outbreak of a false virus to control and own all humanity with their Internet of Things (IoT) connected by wifi to our brains from the vaccines to the Internet of Bodies (IoB), the light is showing us the way to Universal Healing.

My Path to Biomagnetic Healing

My journey towards discovering Biomagnetic Healing began from my involvement with activism beginning in my mid 40's and additionally, from an emotional divorce in my 50's which activated the polio vaccine that both my brother and I received when we were about 8 years young. I have learned that vaccines are designed to stay in your body for Life! and the polio vax lay dormant in me until it was activated through emotional trauma I experienced, according to Dr. Garcia when he diagnosed me. I have since learned that the polio vaccine also was activated with my brother, who died from the polio vaccine at age 38.

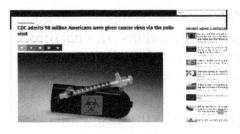

The CDC has now ADMITTED that the **polio vaccine has killed over 98 million people to date**…from the vaccine, not the polio and really caused by DDT used in the farms in the 1950's!!! Once they changed the DDT formula, no more "polio" symptoms, so they sold the vaxxines because they *knew* people would get healthier who had consumed the contaminated DDT. Included in the polio vaccine contained the SV40 monkey virus that induced cancer in people! Thus, we have proof from the CDC themselves that mass genocide was committed on those, like me and my brother, who got the "polio vaccine" sugar cube. My brother is one of these statistics and left 5 children at the age of 38, truth be told.

My true healing came when I broke my back at age 40 that threatened to ruin a pretty good athletic career to that date. Since my family is all Western Medi-Sin indoctrinated with doctor degrees and such, I was forwarded to the top back doc in San Francisco to help me with a severe herniated back that occurred when I popped the S5-L1 vertebrae that caused sever sciatica and pain down my leg like I had never experienced before.

The doctor who saw me was the football team SF 49er's back doctor. He said to me upon his initial examination, "This is one of the worst herniated discs I have ever seen!" (mind you he sees professional football players daily ☺) He diagnosed me and said that I must be in a lot of pain and that the only 'fix' was fused back surgery and I may never get to play sports again, which was my love and passion. However, I may still have pain but not as much.

I asked if yoga, diet, etc. could help me recover in anyway. His reply was, "no, I've been doing this for 20 years now and surgery is the only fix that works for what you have".

Disillusioned, I left his office and called my yogini friend who held a yoga class one day on an island on Lake Shasta. After that one yoga class my body felt rejuvenated and freer. I was much more flexible and not as prone to severe muscle cramping as I had been in the past. She told me to call her yoga teacher friend, go to her classes and just trust her. She also said that most yoga instructors learned to heal themselves from back injuries and such as well, so I would be in good hands. I went regularly to class and began to see improvement slowly but regularly and consistent improvement. Within a couple months I was out of pain! In a few months thereafter, I had a younger body then when I broke my back in the first place! I could play all the athletics I used to and was more agile and more flexible. My mind was clearer and I then practiced yoga and mindful meditation regularly. In addition to my healing, I regularly did physical therapy, changed my diet and paid for a new MRI to show the 49er football physician that I healed myself principally with yoga, physical therapy, change of diet and accupuncture. He refused to see me.

This, after telling me over and over and over in his office that there was *"NO OTHER WAY TO HEAL YOU, JAMIE"* and he repeated over and over, "I've been doing this for 20 years... trust me!" So I proved him wrong, and he didn't want to know. Hippocrites Oath indeed!

As a standard business practice this is also known as "plausible denial". This means if you don't know about it, you can say you never knew, or were aware, of any alternative healing modalities. If he learned there were better, less invasive procedures to get your body back..yet the conflict is personal since "the good doctor" was getting $12 thousand per surgery. Bottom line is that if we can heal ourselves…he is out of income streams, prestige and status as a high degree medic. He has no incentive to look at alternative healing modalities that will affect his earnings. **And why are doctors always "practicing "anyway???**

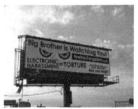

More recently, besides having had a herniated disc at age 40, I have been recently attacked by sophisticated directed energy weapons for my activist work. We are known as "Targeted Individuals or TI's " that are attacked using psychotronic sophisticated weaponry. This is a well-known arm of the US Intelligence and DARPA and beyond arsenal of wireless illness induced torture and pain both physically and emotionally and is highly sophisticated torture technology.

The attacks began on me when I produced a 3 hour long documentary on this very subject titled "Touchless Torture, Target Humanity", back in 2014 and again when I did my 90 + "Paradise Lost" videos on the genocide fires and laser attacks on the innocent people of Paradise, California on November 8th, 2018.

I could feel the laser frequency energy points of entry with directed energy weapons (DEW) on my legs and back while putting the piece together over several months. I could feel the energy enter my heel and then my foot and leg would then swell up while I tried to sleep.

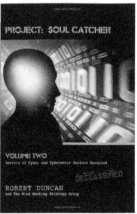

(An excellent book to learn more about Touchless Torture is in a most important book by Dr. Robert Duncan, "Soul Catcher", and is a must read to understand this kind of torture is being planned for us all now and activated through vaccines and 5G).

I have had to readjust my life in how I walked, where I could go, and who I could see. I had extremely limited leg strength or able to walk at a distance. I used to rely on my legs for everything, competing on the World Cup Mogul Skiing, playing Divsion I Tennis, and even riding my bike 200 miles in one day. Yet now my legs were compromised to having two dropped feet and limited control and use of my feet at all. Nothing I tried to heal could alleviate my issues, whether it be yoga, acupuncture, laser therapy, swimming, weightlifting, biofield tuning, massage, mediation, diet change, etc. Nothing got better, nothing helped me. I tried it all but never improved, or if did see improvement, I would rescind back over short period of times to my baseline of issues.

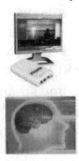

BIOFEEDBACK

IF IT WASN'T SCIENCE IT WOULD BE A MIRACLE

Six years on, a gentleman came up to me at an activist meet up event I was hosting offering to help me with my legs. I was skeptical. A few weeks later he came to my home and conducted a Biomag healing session he had learned from Dr. Goiz on me as I laid out on my bed. He proceeded to place magnets around my body. The session lasted about an hour and I got up and felt no improvement yet thanked him for trying and paid him $200 for his time. He then proceeded with two more sessions with me. The 3rd one I was not with him, but he conducted the healing session some 80 miles away. He told me he placed the magnets for me remotely using a surrogate who came to his house to act as proxy for me, essentially using her body to help heal me. I was skeptical since the first two sessions showed no improvements, but he had me contact several souls he had helped that gave me testimony about their miraculous improvements by this gentleman.

In addition to my leg issues, a year earlier I also had throat issues for over a year, where just swallowing food became very difficult for me at times and I could only drink fluis. Several months earlier, those issues had abated. After a remote session was held for me, my 3rd with this man… I was driving home, after a deep tissue massage, my throat clogged once more anew where I could not swallow. My same symptoms had now come back again and I screamed out, "Noooooooo, not again, he's made me worse, my throat issues are back again, ughhh!".

I then proceeded to go home and make love to the porcelain God, once again, trying to extricate the fluid and small piece of food I tried to digest…that I hoped I was past having these issues….cursing as the throat/swallowing issues had returned and I believed this person had caused it with his magnetic healing work.

Herxheimer Reaction

Or Healing-Crisis Reaction

- The die-off of toxin-producing micro-organisms releases toxins into the body and as one takes treatment to get better, they feel temporarily worse with headache, myalgias, arthralgias, abdomen pain, nausea, vomitting, diarrhea, constipation, brain fog, anxiety, depression, insomnia (described first by German Dr. Karl Herxheimer)
- Herx reactions resolved rapidly in the study using homeopathic & herbal drainage remedies
- Adverse reactions are <u>rare</u> with this natural treatment other than Herxheimer

Copyright MJ Sanders 2009-2019

After several attempts to extricate, I meditated and then said out loud, "All Right!, everyone out NOW!!". I then proceeded to vomit and expel some of the nastiest black goo from my throat into the sink that I had ever seen before. I could not even look at it, since it had such an evil presence to it. I flushed it down the sink immediately.

Within minutes the entire right side of my body opened up and I could breathe like I had not in years. My lungs, my chest and my throat opened where I could breathe freely, like I had not since the first initial throat issues occurred.

The next day I could walk much further without difficulty breathing, without a lot of sweating and I could eat and drink again, without worry. My balance returned and I could breathe much easier and better. It was amazing to experience. This is called a Herxheimer reaction, where the body is expelling the toxic cells in our bodies broken up through the Biomag Healing protocols.

Subsequently, through muscle test scanning, it was found that I had been sprayed with Yersinia Pestis, or the Black Plague, that was delivered through the aerosol spraying chemtrails we see regularly in our skies today. Dr. Garcia also diagnosed me with polio from the vaccine I got when I was 8 that was activated by the emotional trauma of going through my divorce 6 years prior when my leg issues first began. Like most of us, it is not just one symptom, issue or ailment, our maladies involve several and many internal, emotional, terrain and Spiritual toxins in our toxic terrain, food and air.

Biomagnetism deals with the most common pathogens (bacterial, fungal, viral, parasitical) we take in from our terrain, as well as toxicity from vaccines, scars from surgeries and much, much more. Pets shed and mosquito bites are also highly infectious to humans on a regular basis.

Let's Heal the World

So, I then proceeded to learn all I could about biomagnetism through the healer that helped me until he became someone who I could no longer trust or could work with and had to break away…yet I was determined to learn this Biomag healing protocol.

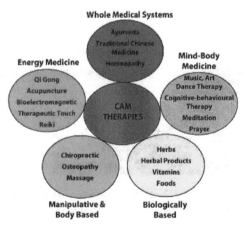

The gentleman that first helped me and had showed me Biomag Healing Protocol had found Biomag healing and it saved his life. He was dying of cancer had lost 1/3rd of his body weight until he learned of Dr. Goiz 's Biomagnetic Polarity healing. He traveled to get this subtle vibrational healing protocol applied to him in a desperate hope to save his life from a BiomagHealer who happened to live within driving distance from him in California. Within 2 month he was diagnosed as cancer free! He then went to study under Dr. Goiz, who resides in Mexico and had helped heal hundreds with this method.

I immediately decided to dedicate my life and learn the Art of Biomag Healing. In April of 2019, I flew to New Jersey and began to learn BiomagHealing from the master himself, Dr. Luis Garcia who was trained under Dr. Goiz.

I learned how magnets were universal energy and how, if we bring our bodies into energetic alignment (homeostasis) and balance of Ph using magnets then pathogens like bacteria, fungus, parasites and virus' can no longer live in our bodies and we attain optimal health.

We are all energetic beings first and foremost, yet western medicine never treats us energetically only take a pill, cut it our and radiate..and then bill…repeat, test, repeat.

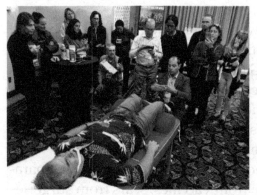

I learned that universal energy is everywhere and through muscle testing all of us can ask questions of from the Universal Spirit guides/angel and get responses and answers in real time. During the five-day intensive I attended Dr. Garcia put me on the massage table and began to scan me for my dropped foot. It was like seeing Michelangelo paint! He began by scanning my body, then using my body as a tool to read what was causing my leg and foot issues.

He would literally ask my body what it needed energetically through muscle testing. He then would apply magnets according to what my body was needing/wanting. Then, he would drill down to find exactly where and what very *specific cells* or nerves, veins, ligaments, bones, etc. that were causing the issue with my dropped foot and then ask for the location to place the two magnets on the body to heal the toxic cells.

Through magnetic polarity of a pulling (black magnet negative) and pushing (red magnet positive) Doc G was attempting to bring my body back into homeostasis, where my body

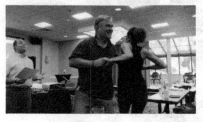

becomes balanced towards an idealized alkalined and acidic state of a PH between 7-7.3. After about 15 pair placements, in less than 1 hour, I got up off the massage table and ran around the convention room in ecstatic joy and grabbed my friend, Paula, and swung and danced with her, like I used to love to do before my feet became an issue with me. Though I was not fully recovered, I found remarkable and profound improvement throughout my lower body and feet. Bottom line, there was noticeable and profound immediate improvement! I felt no pain during the placements, only some tingling, then a surge of energy into my legs as the placements began to take effect in less than 20 minutes time.

I now found what I would be doing for the rest of my life… healing myself and others with Biomagnetic Healing Protocols! Subsequently, I hosted Dr. Garcia, and his lovely wife Juliana, for a 5 day Beyond Biomag Intensive Workshop Training Course in Northern California in October of 2019. Thirty-two souls learned the Art of Self-Healing from Dr. Garcia and were certified thereafter, even as fires swept the area during the weeklong workshop.

As the dark days and months since the Rockefeller engineered Event 201 Planneddemic by the World Economic Council began in November of 2019, we are finding more and more placements to help mitigate injuries due to vaccines, emotional traumas from being locked in and placements to deal with a world in a perpetual induced CRY-us (crisis).

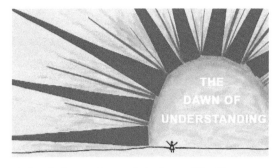

We can now help others at distance as well, remotely. I do not need to be with them or to even know them, for that matter. I just have to ask the Universal Spirits that are helping guide me, if I am *allowed to help this soul or not?* If yes, I then ask the Spirit guides for their assistance to help assist me in finding the correct magnetic placements to help heal another soul with my intention and my placements.

Biomag Healing IS the future of healing for all and we are learning everyday about more and more ways to heal with magnets as well as how to lift effects of vaxxines injuries, that use magnetic principles for their evil desired machinations.

Biomagnetism saves lives, improves lives, and is universal that has no racial, sex or geographical barriers..none! Many of you will find that learning this protocol will change your lives forever more. Tag you're it!

Chapter 1

What is Biomagentism?

Definitions of Health. 10 Golden Rules of Biomagnetism. Effects of Biomagnetism on the Human Body. How Biomagnetism Works. Magnet Polarities. Biomagnetic Scanning.

The power of the magnetic force is one of the most basic powers in nature. We know that magnetism itself was an ingredient in the primordial soup of our Creation event from which this one Universe began. Magnetism is the force that keeps order in all things by attraction. The Laws of Attraction keeps Nature in perpetual balance over vast periods of time, which is also what biomagnetic healings goals are, to bring us back into balance where pathogens can no longer exist and optimal, prolonged healing and wellbeing occurs. Bottom line is that *we don't get old, we get mold!*

> *Importantly, since 1978, the FDA (Food and Drugs Administration) officially recognizes that magnetic energy application has no health risk and accepts the use of it for healing therapeutic purposes. With few exceptions, Biomag Healing only does not effective change the body if magnets are placed improperly. There is nothing to regulate and everyone can use magnets to heal.*

Emotional issues make up most of our physical maladies and this is one of the many reasons why there is no one panacea for everyone at once. Everyone is different to heal, which is why this healing protocol is specific to the individual but can also mitigate common terrain toxicities we all acquire as well. We are each unique but not special. BiomagHealing drills down to each individuals own issues and symptoms to find healing placements and can also heal common maladies we all inherit.

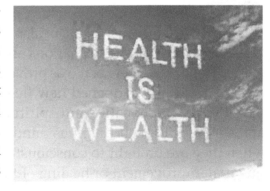

Did you know?

- The microbial signature of each individual, as well as its genome, is unique.
- In every cm2 of our skin, there are about 10,000 bacteria; however, at the hair follicle level in the dermis, there are **1,000,000 bacteria per cm2**.

- Two strains of bacteria are considered to belong to the same species when greater than 70% of their total DNA resembles each other.
- The genetic similarity between a human and a cat is 90%, the human and a mouse 85%, and human with a banana 50%. Man has more than 96% of his DNA equal to that of the chimpanzee.
- Scientists estimate that there are at least 320,000 viruses, just in mammals alone, yet to be discovered.
- If we assume that the 62,305 of the known vertebrate species harbor 58 viruses each, the **number of unknown viruses rises to 3,613,690**. The number rises to 100,939,140 viruses if we include the 1,740,330 known species of vertebrates, invertebrates, plants, lichens, mushrooms, and brown algae. This number does not include viruses of bacteria, archaea, and other single-celled organisms.

Definitions of Health

Allopathic Medicine: Health is the absence of symptoms or disease.

WHO: Health is a state of complete physical, mental, and social well-being, and not only the absence of dis-ease or infirmity.

Claude Bernard: Health depends on the internal balance of living organisms. With pH determining the aspect of such internal balance.

Medical Biomagnetism: Health depends on the organic entropy and that its body's metabolism con-forms to the parameters that are within three tenths of neutral pH toward acidity or alkalinity. But these levels are not static, they are constantly in a state of activity and synergy.

 Bioenergetics is the part of biochemistry concerned with the energy involved in making and breaking of chemical bonds in the molecules found in biological organisms. It can also be defined as the study of energy relationships and energy transformations and transductions in living organisms.

Medical Bioenergetics: It was proven that the power of the mind could replace magnetic energy, and this has opened new fields that allow us to research subjective concepts of psychology, emotionality and spirituality. In understanding its etiology, which often is at the level of the subconscious mind, these often cause pathologies or dysfunctions, but when they are brought to consciousness can be overcome or be forgiven with the consequential improvement or healing of the patient.

Energy healing, *intelligently directs attention* to the origins of illness or concern with the intention to promote healing. As a result, this allows the body's own intelligence to transform the seed of discomfort to its balanced state energetically. The source of the suffering then dissolves as energetic balance is achieved and maintained. The area which it occupied then takes on the form of the original intention of health. Most important, this non-invasive process is easy to learn and get results almost immediately. Healers become conduits, or what I call "Facilitators" to helping another Self-Heal naturally and organically. This keeps the power to heal oneself, with one's self to achieve, and maintain perpetual wellbeing and homeostatic balance. It also keeps the power to heal within one's own possession and not have to rely on men in white coats to 'fix' them.

When I traveled to Tibet they did not have doctors, they had "facilitators". When I asked "why?", they told me because they would never dream of taking the power to heal away from the individual. Heal thyself to be true!

10 GOLDEN RULES OF BIOMAGNETISM
by Doctor Luis Garcia

1. Biomagnetism therapy is a diagnostic and therapeutic procedure.

2. The positive biomagnetic pole is formed by hydrogen ions (H+) and the presence of pathogenic viruses.

3. The negative biomagnetic pole is formed by free radicals and pathogenic bacteria.

4. The magnetic poles are in vibrational and energetic resonance.

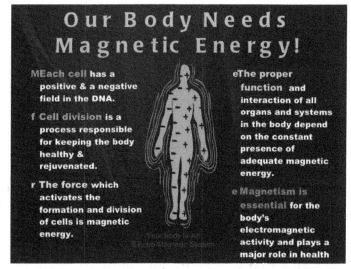

5. The biomagnetic poles are depolarized by the magnetic induction of fields greater than 1000 Gauss.

6. Biomagnetic induction is instantaneous but the charge is exhausted in seconds

7. The ideal magnetic fields for the clinical level of induction are between 5,000 and 20,000 core Gauss.

8. When the biomagnetic poles are impacted, the pathogenic viruses lose their genetic information, and the bacteria its favorable alkaline environment for its metabolism and reproduction.

9. Theoretically, it only requires one impact to eradicate a biomagnetic pair, and it does not reactivate.

10. At the Normal Energetic Level (NEL), pathogenic microorganisms cannot survive, but their metabolites (toxins) may continue to circulate (Ex: Clostridium tetani and tetanus toxins (Tetanospasmin and tetanolysin).

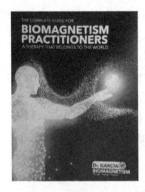

Critical Compliment Book for Most Effective Biomag Healing (usbiomag.com)

In my own opinion, this is the Greatest Medical Book in modern history to date! This book is designed to give you just an introduction to the basics of Biomag Healing Protocol (BHP). This book contains over 300 biomagnetic placements for many injuries and issues, physically and emotionally, we all face today. Western Medi-sin does not even deal with emotional issues causing physical issues, yet, according to Dr. Garcia, emotional issues cause 80% of more physical maladies, which he addresses in this incredible medical healing "Bible". Dr. Garcia has developed hundreds and hundreds of magnetic polarity placements over the 14 years he has focused exclusively on Biomag Healing that are included in this book, including just some of his proprietary scan sheet protocols he himself uses when scanning and diagnosing.

You will need at least one pair of Neodymium N52 magnets to get started with Biomag-Healing. Eventually we will not need magnets as healers, just our energy and our intentions, like Dr. Bruce Rind does with his souls using hands off healing methods that he has proven are very effective. This is where Biomag Healing is heading as well as healing Spiritually, as I discuss further in this book as well.

There are many ways to scan and to find placements for many issues using his "Bible". The full and extremely comprehensive healing protocol Dr. Garcia has developed regularly produces repeated miracle healing with those he works with as documented in Appendix III under "Testimonials".

You may also want to get the what I call the "Scriptures" binder of charts and scan protocols that will be in the follow up book to compliment the Biomag Practitioners, which I offer for sale online. This will help guide, as well as develop, your own personal placement charts as we are all unicorns and snowflakes with our own personal issues. You can order the updated "Scriptures" book at Biomaghealer.com which includes updates for new placements found for dealing with all the mass inoculations by the varying drug manufactures.

Effects Of Magnetic Forces On the Human Body

1. When a magnet is applied to the human body, the passage of magnetic waves through the tissues produces an increase in temperature due to the impact of electrons on the cells of the body. The impacts are very effective in reducing pain and swelling in the muscles, etc.

2. Blood activity is accelerated while the calcium and cholesterol deposits in the blood are diminished. Materials adhered to the inner side of the veins, which cause high

blood pressure, decrease, and tend to fade. The blood is cleansed, and circulation is increased. The activities of the heart are facilitated, and the pain disappears.

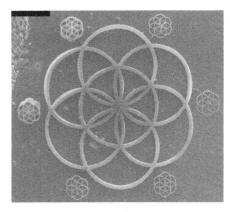

3. The autonomy functions of the nerves are normalized in such a way that the internal organs recover their own function.

4. Magnetic waves penetrate the skin, fatty tissues, and bones, invigorating the organs. The result is greater resistance to diseases.

Although state-of-the-art American medicine uses techniques to monitor magnetic fields, such as electrocardiograms, electroencephalograms, and magnetic resonance imaging (MRI's), it has not taken other forms of magnetic healing modalities seriously. More and more medical studies, however, are confirming the value of the magnetic approach. Now awareness of this modality is filtering down to the general public, as increasing numbers of people are sleeping on magnetic beds at night and wearing small magnets during the day for greater energy, preventive purposes, and healing.

Magnetism is both leading-edge science and traditional "healing protocol" that has been used by the Chinese for 5,000 years. Since then, many cultures have tried magnets with varying results. It is said that Cleopatra slept on a lode stone (natural magnet) to sleep on at night that successfully retained her youth and beauty. Paracelsus, a scientist in the late 1400's, used them successfully with seizures and many other illnesses. More recently, dual polarity magnets have proven to be an effective healing protocol for most diseases.

Biomagnetism is a revolutionary, scientific and therapeutic approach to wellness that differs from traditional medicine, homeopathy, herbs and natural therapies. It is perfectly compatible with any other traditional or alternative modality. This non-invasive protocol is an internationally practiced health approach that strives to attain bio-energetic balance in the human body; the state of natural health known as "homeostasis".

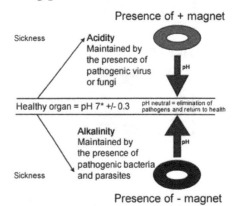

It involves the precise and proper (North/South polarity) placement of special high field strength magnets over very specific areas of the body, to support regulation of pH in these very areas. By maintaining adequate pH, homeostasis may be reestablished so that the body can heal itself. This therapy stimulates normal immune system function, increased circulation and oxygenation, normalizing response to inflammation and many more positive effects on our bodies.

The measurement of pH aims to determine the concentration of hydrogen ions present in a solution. Due to its diminutiveness, hydrogen ions have great mobility and a huge capacity for reaction. H+ ions, are formed throughout the aqueous solutions by the dissociation of water molecules. The H+ concentration in acid substances is greater than in neutral pure water and is lower in bases or alkaline substances. Salts, although in principle considered balanced by the union of an acid and a base in its formation, are frequently not sufficiently compensated for their opposites, so in their clinical behavior usually resemble the acidic or basic element predominantly in it.

Biomagnetism involves placement of special high field strength magnets over very specific areas of the body, to support regulation of pH in these very areas. By maintaining adequate pH, homeostasis may be reestablished so that the body can heal itself.

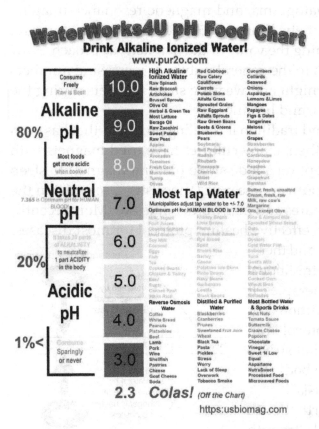

What Is the Importance of pH Balance?

The pH scale goes from 0 to 14, with 7 being neutral. Below 7 is acidic and above 7 is alkaline. Arterial and venous blood must maintain a slightly alkaline pH: arterial blood pH = 7.41 and venous blood pH = 7.36. Because the normal pH of arterial blood is 7.41, this has given rise to a variety of approaches based on increasing the alkalinity of the tissues, such as a vegetarian diet, the drinking of fresh fruit and vegetable juices, and dietary supplementation with alkaline minerals to maintain body pH. Although these strategies help maintain pH, they may not be enough in today's harsh environment.

It is believed that pH imbalances may ultimately accumulate and combine to allow the development of Biomagnetic Pair studies that detects, classifies, measures and allows the correction of pH imbalances in living organisms. By reestablishing the natural pH balance of the body, different microorganisms such as virus, fungi, bacteria and parasites can be kept under control by our renewed natural defenses. For example, when you take a fish out of water, it can no longer survive in that new environment no matter how much oxygen or light is available. All fish need water to survive but some need saltwater, whereas others need freshwater. Everyone who has had an aquarium or pool knows of the importance of pH balance in the water. We are no different. Our body is made up of over 75% water and has a very specific pH balance that it needs to maintain if we are to remain healthy! If we reestablish our body's natural pH balance in our liver, lungs, pancreas, kidneys, muscles, joints, stomach, small intestine, large intestine, etc., then these organs may begin working correctly again. The old saying, "You are what you eat" holds true. If we eat acid-producing foods, then our bodies will shift towards a more acidic pH. More acidic pH is believed to promote inflammation and chronic conditions such as cancer, among

How does Biomagnetism Work?

The penetration value is how deep into the tissue the magnetic effect penetrates. It is very simple – if there is a deep tissue condition, the magnet must be strong enough to penetrate the energy to stimulate the cells correctly. Remember that the effect of the magnets is an all or nothing scenario. The magnets are either 100% effective, or they do no harm = 0% effective. This is also why if you incorrectly place magnets, you will not do any harm yet simply will not get desired the desired effect you intend to receive from that placement.

All Biomagnetic healing magnets are designed to specifically reach the required A-Z penetration values. After a quarter of a century of development, you can be assured the magnetic power used in this energy healing and has been designed for the proper pene-

tration values to help the body heal rapidly – whether you have pain, chronic illness or an acute condition. The radical pair mechanism is the favored hypothesis for explaining biological effects of weak magnetic fields, such as animal magneto -reception and possible adverse health effects. To date, however, there is no direct experimental evidence for magnetic effects on radical pair reactions in cells, the fundamental building blocks of living systems. In the living cells of animals with magnetoreception, proteins called cryptochromes are thought to be the molecules

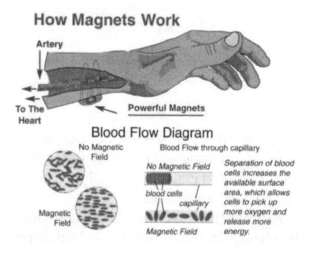

that undergo this radical pair mechanism. And now, researchers at the University of Tokyo have observed cryptochromes responding to magnetic fields for the first time.

The discovery of the electron led to the use of electricity as the primal force over magnetism at the end of the 19th century declaring that everything is partially electric in nature, *thereby excluding magnetism as a force of power*. Electrons also have a property called "spin". In a radical pair, the spins of the two solo electrons are linked – they can either spin together or in opposite directions. These two states have different chemical properties, the radical pair can flip between them, *and the angle of the Earth's magnetic field can influence these flips*. In doing so, it can affect the outcome or the speed of chemical reactions involving the radical pair. This is one of the ways in which the Earth's magnetic field can affect living cells. It explains why the magnetic sense of animals like birds is tied to vision – after all, cryptochrome is found in the eye, and it's converted into a radical pair by light.

North (Negative) Pole ~ Black *PullinGGg/Attraction* ~ Female Principle
South (Positive) Pole ~ Red *Pushing/Repulsion* ~ Male Principle

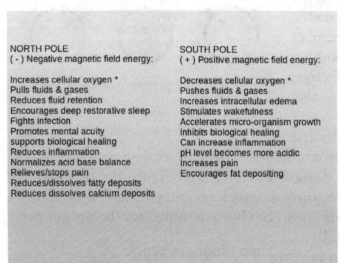

NORTH POLE
(-) Negative magnetic field energy:

Increases cellular oxygen *
Pulls fluids & gases
Reduces fluid retention
Encourages deep restorative sleep
Fights infection
Promotes mental acuity
supports biological healing
Reduces inflammation
Normalizes acid base balance
Relieves/stops pain
Reduces/dissolves fatty deposits
Reduces dissolves calcium deposits

SOUTH POLE
(+) Positive magnetic field energy:

Decreases cellular oxygen *
Pushes fluids & gases
Increases intracellular edema
Stimulates wakefulness
Accelerates micro-organism growth
Inhibits biological healing
Can increase inflammation
pH level becomes more acidic
Increases pain
Encourages fat depositing

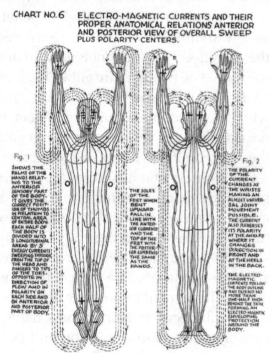

CHART NO.6 ELECTRO-MAGNETIC CURRENTS AND THEIR PROPER ANATOMICAL RELATIONS ANTERIOR AND POSTERIOR VIEW OF OVERALL SWEEP PLUS POLARITY CENTERS.

A 1997 study at Baylor College of Medicine concluded permanent magnets reduce pain in post-polio patients. The results of that study were heralded in newspapers throughout the country, most notably in a Jan. 6, 1999, story in The New York Times.

Around the same time, national magazines reported on the growing use of magnets by champion senior golfers and other professional athletes to relieve pain, resulting in an explosion of magnetic jewelry and other magnetic items for therapeutic use. https://pubmed.ncbi.nlm.nih.gov/9365349/

Though studies by the Medical Mafia are few and far between, another study of using magnets to heal was conducted by the NIH in 2017, titled, "Biomagnetic Pair Therapy and Typhoid Fever: A Pilot Study"

Results: *Most of the participants (10 of 13) retested as negative, and all patients reported symptomatic clinical improvement. Conclusions:* **As a significant majority of participants demonstrated clearing of their S. typhi after BPT**, *this technique should be studied further in larger trials for its efficacy in treating typhoid fever.* https://pubmed.ncbi.nlm.nih.gov/29067141/

The only study to date on alleviating cancer with magnets was published in the September 1990 issue of the "Journal of the National Medical Association." Scientists took petri dishes full of cancer cells and put them in either the biomagnetic north pole end of a magnetic resonance imaging facility or the biomagnetic south pole end. In three weeks, the petri dishes in the north pole end exhibited a dramatic decrease in cell growth, which is what you what you want to see with cancer cells. The dishes in the south end exhibited a slight, but detectable, increase in the rate of cell growth. However, subsequent experiments have proven that magnetic placements can mitigate, arrest and eliminate cancer cells.

This is an image of how science is using magnets to attract cancer cells to lift the cancer from bodies. The same principles apply with BiomagHealing but without the injections. It should be noted that today, magnetic therapy is well established in other countries, such as South America, Mexico, Japan, China, India, Austria, and Germany. In the US you will be sued and fined for using words like "remedy", "cure", "improve" and "restore". I cover more

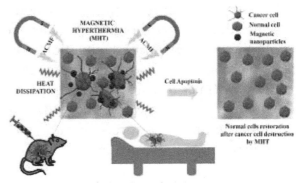

of this legalese in Appendix VI "Setting Up Your Biomag Business".

(Note: the reason for the absurd definitions here is because we live on a Flat plane, so this is astronomers heliocentric non-sensical explanation.)

The North Pole is NOT magnetic North since the Earths' core is magnetic and the South Pole is really the positively charged Antarctic Circle, much like how a speaker works.

1. The actual north pole of the magnet is defined as the north-GEOGRAPHIC seeking pole, and this is because that is where the Earth's magnetic SOUTH pole is.

2. The actual south pole of the magnet is defined as the south-GEOGRAPHIC seeking pole, and this is because that is where the Earth's magnetic NORTH pole is.

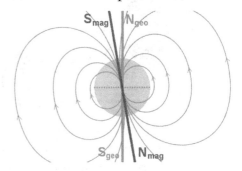

3. The earth's magnetic NORTH POLE is in the south (geographically), and the earth's magnetic SOUTH POLE is in the north (geographically).

The **Geographic North Pole** & Magnetic South Pole decreases the development of pathogens and increases the defenses against them. Increases the oxygenation of tissues to decrease inflammation and edema. Alkalizes the ground reducing the symptoms of acidic conditions. You can dispel headaches in a few minutes. It can dissolve crystals of various types and reduces the calcium deposits in arthritic joints. Helps to dissolve blood clots. It reduces organ hyperactivity, as well as the activity of proteins. It reduces the bleeding of wounds and light hemorrhages.

The **Geographic South Pole** and Magnetic North Pole can increase organ activity, stimulating its functions. Increases the development of live tissues. Accelerates the metabolic processes. Opens clogged or hardened ducts due to increased flexibility (capillaries, veins, arteries). Strengthens heart function and can produce tachycardias. Faster growth of normal tissues. Resolution of fractures 3-5 times faster.

There are no real contra indications to receiving biomagnetism, just precautions. Biomagnetism may be applied during pregnancy. An experienced energy healer will know to ask whether the therapy should be best applied for the mother or baby or both and how to apply the magnets for each situation. Souls with a history of epilepsy may also benefit from Biomagnetism and must understand that when toxins are being released from the body, sometimes a detox reaction may occur whereby there is a temporary increase in inflammation that may affect the soul temporarily. Think about working out again for the first time, your muscles are sore, not strong yet, because it mst go through a short period of adjustment to the new stimuli.

Biomagnetic Diagnosing

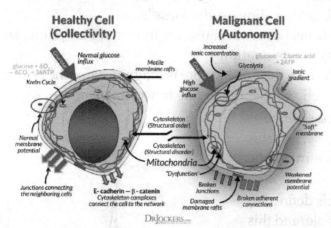

The measurement of the biomagnetic poles, to date, is qualitative and indirect. The identification of a biomagnetic pair is indicative of a pathology. It is advisable to carry out the diagnosis with the north or negative pole since they are more extensive and unique, while the positive magnetic pole can occasionally establish resonance with two or more negative poles. The left hemi-body usually remains fixed in its dimensions, since the heartbeat depolarizes it every second, while the right is the one that stretches or contracts, with which we can qualitatively measure the altered organ. 90% of Magnets are placed on the right side of the body *to pull* us back into balance from being *pushed out* of balance, in simple terms.

Diagnosing can come through muscle testing, hands on healing, using a dowser or just by intuition but there always needs to have a pair for polarity to bring the body back into ideal homestasis.

It is magnetism, along with cold and hot plasma fields omnipresent energies, that keeps the sun and the moon in rotation above us that create our seasons. The magnetism maintains perpetual motion as well as distance when the positive and negative energy fields are activated by the salt water, just like a battery. Birds use magnetism to navigate, so do ships, and every computer, power generator and moving vehicle would not operate without magnets. We never hear about magnetism, only EL-ectricity from the El-ite who wish to El-liminate the Peep-El through mass innocul-ations we now are very aware, if you are awake and paying attention. So how is it that EL-ectricity is so well known, yet magnetism, though it is essential for all life and is the world's greatest healer, is unknown by the masses and unrecognized by Wester Med-i-sin?

A: By design, by design. For profit first and only is Big pHarma's only purpose to exist as well as to keep all willfully ignorant and in ill-health for maximizing profits and shareholder value. That's it! The medical Profess-sin model is about business only! It does not care about you, your children or your wellbeing, just profits, only profits and to keep you sick and designs its drugs to never cure, in fact you cannot even use the word 'cure' with the medical mafia.

Magnets are *Free energy, Universal and Can Heal* and Protect All…the basic principles for the Femine Devine. "El" is the male principal represented by Toth, Apollo, Jesus Christ, etc. Electricity is not created, it is transferred. The male cannot create only seed.

Men cannot bear and give life, only a woman can. A woman just needs a frozen male seed, not the male to create life. Men cannot 'bear fruit', only Whoa Man can! Magnetism is the Feminine Devine reincarnating now through Biomagnetic Healing, how cool is that? Nurture/Nature creating health and well-being for all who wish it. Free and accessible to heal and to balance a very out of balance world today.

Magnet. **Mag**ic. **Mag**nificent. **Mag**nanomous. **Mag**ma **Mag**us. **Mag**i. **Mag**nify. **Mag**istrate. Mary **Mag**delena. i**Mag**ine.

Why are all these powerful words start with "**Mag**"? Because they all refer to something much greater than just one, or just us! The Laws of Attraction which holds the duality of all life together, as the male Law of Repulsion wars and pushes away as it tries to dominate, like it has for the past thousand years and more. The end of the male dominance is over now as the Feminine Devine takes her thrown as Lourdess of healing and the life creating forces of Nature.

The law of Attraction is what brings two opposites together. Like minded magnets are repelled by their sameness, our Universe is literally, and figuratively, an entire field in balance and polarity of opposites that are attracted to one another in perpetual motion.

It is the Feminine Devine principle of Creation that has been denied to this day as being heretical as declared by the Men in Black Catholic Order of the Vatican and above to be evil to hide the power of Attraction. The primarily male hierarchy, who have kept the Feminine Devine buried while debasing the status of women in general, wish to keep all from knowing their true cosmic place in this duality of Creations of male/female, ying/ yang, electricity/magnetism, creation/dissolution, mind/matter, etc.

The dark Satanic religious zealots who wish to own all souls forever, The Vatican and the Catholic church, state that Mary was a Charlatan and a whore. Additionally, "THE KJV Bible", written by a King and final edited by Sir Francis Bacon, the Founder of Freemasonry as well as just one of just hundreds of known Bib-els.. states that the first woman, Eve, was created by a rib of Adam…a cheaper cut. It was Eve who ate the apple and ruined it for all. It was the woman who ruined it for the Man. We are called hue-Men, per-Sons, and pay money for Fee-males. Women were not even allowed to vote or have equal status just several decades previous. The powers that should not be have successfully suppressed the Femine Devine beginning with changing to the Roman Catholic Gregorian calendar from the more accurate Moon calendar previous that most Natives went by with 13 months.

Chapter 2

Let's Heal the World

What Can Biomagnetism Heal?

Please visit **www.Biomaghealer.com** to order books, water purifiers, magnets, etc. as well as you can download zoom webinars to learn the principles of self-healing with online webinars and workshops that compliment this book to learn how to effectively place magnets for these issues and many, many more.

Here are just a few healing results from magnets from Gary Null's book *"Healing With Magnets"*.

Aging. Magnets activate life-promoting enzymatic activity which, in turn, encourages normal cell division. This creates a healthier organism and may then slow down the aging process. Several studies on animals show magnetic therapy to increase lifespan. In order to balance the energy of the organs and glands throughout the body, it has been suggested that one apply magnetic fields to the whole body. Sleeping on a magnetic bed is an excellent way to accomplish this. Drinking magnetized water is another good habit to get into. Additionally, injured or weak areas of the body can be strengthened by applying magnets to these specific sites.

Relief from Pain and Discomfort. The most common use of magnetic fields is in the treatment of pain, with reports of successful treatment in a wide variety of conditions, including arthritis, rheumatism, fibromyalgia, back pain, headaches, muscle sprains and strains, joint pain, tendonitis, shoulder pain, carpal tunnel syndrome, and torn ligaments. A noteworthy American double-blind, placebo-controlled study on the effects of static magnets on the treatment of arthritis was recently published in the ®MDBR "Journal of Rheumatology®MDNM" (November 1997, p. 1200). The study confirms the effectiveness of magnets in relieving the pain of arthritis. Another scientific study of similar rigor is being carried out by Dr. Zimmerman and is looking at the effects of fixed magnets on low back pain. There is good reason to expect confirmation of what users have been claiming for years--that magnets are an excellent aid to pain relief. To understand how magnets work to alleviate pain it may help to look at pain mechanisms in the body.

Pain is transmitted along nerve cells as an electric signal. While quiescent, the nerve has a small charge of about -70 mV. A pain signal depolarizes a cell. Magnets appear to raise

23

the depolarization potential of the cell so that the signal is blocked from depolarization, in effect, blocking the pain. Furthermore, the ability of the nerve to send pain is slowed by a magnetic field. These phenomena can aid in the relief of pain throughout the body. Pain relief may be enhanced when a magnet's negative pole is placed over certain acupuncture meridians. Research and clinical experience show that magnets increase energy (qi) along these points.

The combination of therapies works synergistically so that their combined effects are greater than the sum of their effects would be if they were used separately. In addition, acupuncturists like magnets because they are painless and allow the treatment to continue long after a visit. Reduction of Inflammation and Improved Circulation. Injured tissue emits a positive charge; placing the negative pole of a magnet over the area appears to restore a natural balance in the following way: The magnet improves circulation, allowing blood vessels to dilate and bring a greater volume of blood flow to the injured area.

This helps to bring in natural healers and to remove the toxic byproducts of inflammation--bradykinens, prostaglandins, and histamines--all of which contribute to inflammation and pain. Thus, pain and inflammation are diminished, and tissue healing is stimulated. Antimicrobial Effects Magnetic therapy can help the body ward off such microbial invaders as viruses, bacteria, and fungi. It achieves this, in part, by increasing immune function through the oxygenation of white corpuscles, an important part of the immune system's arsenal. A magnetic field can also function like an antibiotic by lowering acidity, with the result that microorganisms have a more difficult time surviving. In addition, hormonal production is regulated, altering enzymatic activity and biochemical messengers of the immune system.

For example, the pineal gland is one large electromagnetic entity. The net effect is to augment the body's natural ability to resist a variety of germs.

Stress Reduction. The recent discovery of magnetite in the cells of the brain helps explain the calming effect of biomagnetic healing. A magnetic field applied to the head calms as well as induces a hypnotic sleeping effect on the brain by stimulating the hormone melatonin. Melatonin is known to be anti-stressful, producing a sedating effect in insomniacs. This finding has led to the manufacture of magnetic pillows and pads designed to provide a sound and restful sleep. A person can then awaken with more energy and fewer aches and pains. Correction of Central Nervous System Disorders Dr. William Philpott claims that biomagnetic healing can help central nervous system disorders. He states that such symptoms as hallucinations, delusions, seizures, and panic can be alleviated through biomagnetic therapy without disrupting the patient's mental alertness and orientation. Also, a magnetic field may reduce the need for tranquilizers and antidepressants. Magnets have been used as well to stop epileptic seizures.

Energy Enhancement. Biomagnetic therapy is known to increase general well-being by enhancing energy. The normal polarization of a positively charged nucleus with a negatively charged outer membrane permits a cell to function as a healthy entity. However, as the cell performs its daily functions, it becomes depolarized. Depolarized cells equal a tired person. It is believed that magnetic energy can penetrate all facets of the human body and reach every cell. That translates to greater energy and vitality throughout the body as a whole. Consequently, supplemental biomagnetic therapy can help the body revitalize. One normally revitalizes biological energy during sleep. This can be enhanced by sleeping in a magnetic field. Then, anabolic hormones, such as melatonin and DHEA, are made. Melatonin, made by the pineal gland, is a master hormone controlling the entire energy system.

Quicker Healing. The medical community has known for years that pulsed biomagnetic therapy promotes the healing process, particularly of bone fractures. For over 40 years, many doctors have used pulsed biomagnetic therapy to treat fractures and have had a high rate of success. Several magnetic instruments have already been FDA-approved and sanctioned for both safety and therapeutic implications. The success of this therapy is attributed, in part, to it facilitating the migration of calcium ions and osteoblasts to heal broken bones in less than the usual time. In addition, the migration of calcium occurs away from joints to reduce painful arthritic joint inflammation. The result is the noninvasive promotion of natural healing, without the use of unnatural chemicals and drugs. Adequate magnetic energy also softens or eliminates scar tissue formed during the healing process. Some doctors put magnets into the dressings over fractures. In fact, one veterinarian I know, who broke his ankle after falling from a horse, reported following this strategy on himself.

Increased Athletic Endurance and Performance. For years, magnetic therapy has been used around the world on racehorses to heal injuries and enhance performance. Doug Hannum, owner of the Equine Therapy Center in Camden, South Carolina, employs magnetic blankets along with other natural healing modalities on animals, and professional riders, such as five-time Olympian Bruce Davidson and world championship rider Dorothy Trapp, ship their steeds to Hannum for therapy. Stunning successes with animals have prompted professional athletes to use magnets. The Russians may have been the first in recent athletic history to have adapted magnetic therapy to foster greater athletic strength and achievement. Today, many notable American athletes embrace this technology as well. Denver Bronco linebacker Bill Romanowski revitalized his aching body by sleeping on a magnetic mattress pad. Yankee pitcher Irabu plays with dozens of magnets stuck to his body. Top golfer Jim Colbert endorses magnets. And professional football player Steve Atwinter, a seven-time pro-bowler, says, "I am not waiting for scientists to bless it. I only know it works." Even high schools are turning to magnetic therapy to improve athletic performance. Although the effect of increased endurance and performance is known, the cause is not definitively understood. It is felt that magnetic energy warms up the muscles and joints so that performance is increased. At least as important, serious injuries are reduced. In addition, it is known that magnetic energy increases blood flow to the muscles, thereby increasing strength at these work sites.

Specific Uses. In addition to its general benefits, biomagnetic healing may help a variety of specific conditions. This is not to say that magnets will cure absolutely, irreversibly, and indefinitely. How much good they do vary from person to person and depends upon such factors as the depth of the problem, how long the condition has been in existence, and how strong the magnet is.

Also, when using magnets for chronic longstanding conditions, where the tissues have not been getting adequate blood flow, you may at first get an exacerbation of symptoms. Some people call this a healing crisis. The discomfort usually passes in 24 to 48 hours.

Emotional Healing. The resulting emotional issues associated with being lockdown in place for well over a year now IS real and is having severe effects on all. Biomagnetism can help greatly with brain fog, depression, anxiety, loss, fear, etc.

Spiritual Clearing. This is the next level to optimal Biomag healing protocols is to remove and transform, not translocate, spiritual demons affecting and effecting our health today. As I explain in further detail there are physical demons and emotional demons that are associated with every single issue we all have. To locate and to remove them is another key to full healing and wellbeing.

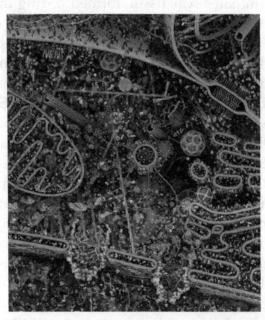

Spectronic Microscope Imagery of a Single Cell

Chapter 3

Let's Heal the World ~ Applied Biomagnetic Healing

Methods of Muscle Testing. Session Work ~ Let's Begin to Heal. Remote Healing at a Distance
Please go to Biomaghealer on You Tube to watch tutorial on how to learn to muscle test…(https://youtu.be/YGRJoJMnuVc).

Methods of Muscle Testing

Chiropractors often use one form of muscle testing but there are over a dozen techniques, or you can develop your own to allow Spiritual energy to work through you.

Getting Started

Relax, Clear the Mind, Breathe

Use one of the methods below to begin and begin muscle scanning with no expectations of outcome. Begin with a clear mind.

1. Begin movement and stop to get even baseline indicator, (i.e. fingers even, thumbs even, arms equal length, etc.) so they are even and aligned.

2. Start movement of hands or fingers then stop after asking the first question and see if baseline has moved on either digit or one arm is longer than another. On 2nd question do the same. If standing, your body will likely sway forward or back after the question is asked.

3. Begin by moving digits, or arms at side, or body still and command the question to your indicators "Show me a Yes!" either out loud of silently, it makes no difference.

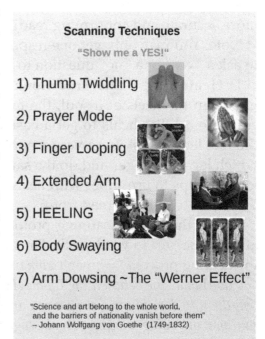

Scanning Techniques

"Show me a YES!"

1) Thumb Twiddling

2) Prayer Mode

3) Finger Looping

4) Extended Arm

5) HEELING

6) Body Swaying

7) Arm Dowsing ~The "Werner Effect"

"Science and art belong to the whole world, and the barriers of nationality vanish before them" – Johann Wolfgang von Goethe (1749-1832)

4. Stop movement and see if one digit has moved relative to another. You will likely see that one finger, thumb, leg, arm, hand, etc. has moved higher, or more forward than another. If you get movement, this confirms a "Yes" for your muscle testing. If standing, you will feel your body move forward or move backwards.

5. Set your baseline again and clear your mind once more. Now move your digits and command, "Show me a No!" and see if your body sways the other way or the other digit moved longer. If so, this is your "No" indicator.

6. Continue asking 'yes' and 'no' questions and observe your own muscle testing response. Everyone has different methods and different degrees of response but the more you work with this energy, the better the responses become over time. You can ask questions like, "Is my name so and so?" and see a response, then ask is my name "a no response" and observe and see if the other digit moves. This will show, and confirm, that your muscle testing responses are now available to you.

THE MORE YOU PRACTICE, the more active your muscle testing will become. In addition, as your muscle testing advances you will notice on some scans your digit will get significantly longer, or just a small movement. This can be and indicator of severity of issue or symptom. A big movement, big issues, small movement, not so much.

Now try the other techniques and see if you get any responses. (You will need another person to do the leg testing). By having various techniques of muscle testing you will be able to confirm, confirm and confirm your readings and well as provide you with ever more accurate and confirming readings and scans of your souls.

Note: You may only get one response to start, which is fine. All you need is to be able to ask a "yes" or a "no" question to be able to muscle scan successfully.

1) **Hea(e)ling ~ The Traditional Method** ~ By lining up the heels of a soul, the faciliatory gently cups the achilles heals to get a baseline reading of the feet length. Ask for a yes response and note if/which leg gets longer and do the same for the other leg. (It helps to use shoes with heals that can give a definitive baseline to read from).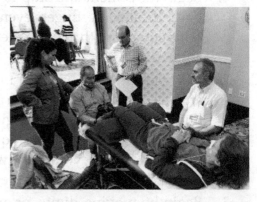

This is the classic scanning protocol but requires another person to work with. Dr. Garcia describes the healing process: "*Through a binary (extension-contraction) dialogue between the BiomagHealer and bodily cells, feet respond by either shorting or lengthening depending of the particular polarity of the soul you are to get a reading from. Lay the soul you are going to scan on a massage table or bed, and have their feet dangle off the end right above the ankles.*

Now see if their heels are even at the bottom so you get a baseline indicator to work with. When even, begin the protocol scanning questions above. You do not need to see large movement, just noticeable change. Over time you will then be able to feel the legs shift when you ask questions. The therapy consists in its own diagnostic tool by placing the negative magnet on any of the hundreds of points in the body that make up the biomagnetic-pairs. If the body gives a reaction it means, there is a pathological problem. This will happen when the right leg shrinks, which can easily be detected by comparing the edge of the two heels.

The BiomagHealer places a magnet on a point, for example the thyroid, and then checks the length of the feet. If the right leg shrinks, then the practitioner knows that there is a problem and will place the other magnet in the corresponding bio-magnetic pair. In the case of the thyroid it is the back of the head, which according to Dr. Goiz, identifies a meningitis infection. If, after placing the second magnet, the legs return to equal lengths, the practitioner knows that a bio-magnetic pair that needed correction has been identified and will leave the magnets in place for about 15 minutes. In this short time the problem is supposed to be corrected – in this case, the meningitis virus has been eliminated. Thus, in this point-by-point way, the whole body is scanned to detect specific viruses, bacteria, fungi and parasites that – according to Dr. Goiz – find their alkaline or acid niches to survive and, through a resonance effect, cause almost all diseases".

2) **Prayer Mode** ~ Put your hands in prayer and hold near eye level. Look to see if your two middle fingers are even at the top of your fingers. If not make them even. Now open and close your hands outward while keeping your palms at the base together. Fingers away and together again forming a "V" at the base. You can even clap make a clapping sound with your hands. Stop again and see if your middle fingers are even. Now go through the question tree above and see if you get any responses. You can even do this with your eyes closed as not to influence finger movement. Remember to clear the mind and clear any expectations.

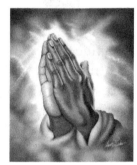

3) **Thumb Twiddling** ~ This was the first muscle scanning technique that worked for me. From the prayer position above, fold your fingernails inwards on each other where your knuckles are touching and your two thumbs facing you. Now see if your thumbs are even. If not, make them even. Twiddle, twiddle, twiddle your fingers. Out and back or forward and back does not matter. Relax and clear your mind. Now when twiddling, ask the 'yes', then the 'no' questions and see if one thumb, or the other, gets longer. Note which digit moves to 'yes', and 'no', if at all.

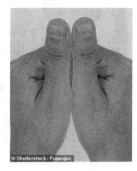

4) **Finger Gating** ~ Take one hand and touch your pinky finger with your index figure creating a loop. Touch your finger and thumb together lightly. With your other hand put

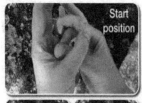
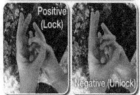

your index and thumb together and stick inside 'gate' on other hand. (It does not matter which hand you use). With the finger inside the 'gate' loop of the other hand ask a question and try and "open the gate" by moving your inside index finger up to move the "gate" open. This is subtle action, so make sure you are relaxed. If you get an answer, your 'gate' loop will open. With me, I get a "yes" answer when the gate opens and a "no" when I find that it is more resistant to opening the 'gate'. Either way will work. You are only looking to find a response, be it a "yes" or a "no" answer.

5) Finger Crossing ~ The X Factor

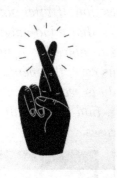

This method is my go to now since I can do muscle testing with just one hand and can go very fast now. When first testing this method one finger will cross over the other and the other response will be no movement. Allow your fingers to move and cross if they want to.

Simply hold up your index and 2nd finger and twiddle them. Ask the questions and see if one finger wants to cross over the other. It is more subtle than the other techniques. One answer will be the fingers stay aligned like the number 11 and the other crosses over the other as shown in the image. You only need one response to be effective and you can ask your fingers to switch…make the "yes" cross over instead of the "no" answer. At first you will resist letting your fingers to cross….just let it happen and soon you will be able to use either and muscle test without anyone even knowing you are doing it.

(At first my "no" was crossed fingers and then I instructed my fingers for the crossing to be my "yes" and now my "yes" is a crossed finger and my "no" is even).

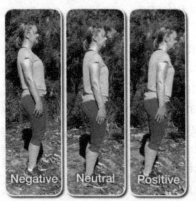

6) Sway Testing ~ Stand with your feet comfortably underneath you and clear your mind and close your eyes (if you can stay still). Then asks the questions and note if a "yes' moves your body forward or backward and a "no" response the opposite. Others can see you move from the side. Someone can watch your body movement from the side as well to see if you've swayed back or forwards.

7) Arm Testing ~ Put both arms at your side, relax your shoulders while standing up. Put your arms out at shoulder level and put your hand together in a light fist. Note if your arms are the same length at the end of your knuckles, if not make them even. Now drop your arms, relax and ask a question while bringing your arms back up and see if one arm has gotten longer than another in response.

8) **Dowsing**. Many empaths use dowsing methods to find answers to questions, others develop their own way of asking the Universe questions that work for them and still others just 'feel' the answer (clairsentient) or 'hear' a voice in their head (clairaudient) or just 'know' the answer (clairvoyant). Whatever works best for you.

I cannot emphasize enough what a powerful tool this is for all. Younger generations and children tend to get results easier than some adults because they are still connected to Source. You can use this to question everything from 'should I eat this food' to "what time will he show up" to "am I in danger if I do this".

The more direct the question, the more direct the answer. Remember you are asking the Universe to give you answers and guidance, so it is important to be very, very specific with your intentions and your questions. As one example I learned was when I asked, "will this placement help this soul?" I would get a yes but get no results from the session. Then I learned to ask, "will this placement help this soul…*Today!* The lesson I learned was to be very specific with your questions. The reason is that I want to do placements that will help now, not in the future time frame when more placements will be used. You can also ask the same question with a 'yes' and 'no' to confirm. "Are there any more placements needed here"? "No". Then ask, "Are you sure" and get a "Yes" response to show your fingers are reacting to your inquiries. I do this with every placement to confirm, confirm, confirm.

Think if everyone learned muscle testing aka the "Ultimate b.s. Detector!" we would have instant peace in the world.

Session Work ~ Let's Begin
Focus, Clear Mind and Setting Intention

(Appendix I-II lays out the format and details of how to go through a session of BiomagHealing with an individual.)

First set out your own intentions for helping this soul with magnets today. Are you doing a full scan? Or dealing with their issues, symptoms and pain? or need to address emotional issues?

Is this a remote session or in person? Are you going to prescan before you meet them, or wait until you see them? Do you have a personal emotional attachment you need to clear in yourself to help heal the soul most effectively? How much time do we need today? How many magnets can I place per session?

A Biomag Healing Session studies, detects, classifies, measures and allows the correction of pH imbalances in living organisms. By reestablishing the natural pH balance of the body, different microorganisms such as virus, fungi, bacteria and parasites can be kept under control by our renewed natural defenses. Once our body is brought back to homeostasis diseases, pathogens and toxicities in our environment can be mitigated, balanced and/or eliminated from our bodies.

There are literally hundreds of ways to Biomag Heal but it all begins with setting intention! The very first question when beginning the protocol of Biomag Healing is, "Can I help this person today with placing magnets"? If you get a "yes" answer with your muscle testing, then proceed, if "no", then you are not supposed to do any placements for them that day, yet ask again in the future and you may get a different response.

Note: It is very important to take before and after pictures and testimonies to chronicle, validate and improvements and progression

Session Work with Souls

Primary is to set out your expectations with those you are attempting to help with their issues. Identify that you are a facilitator and that you are assisting them but they will be activating the energy to heal with their bodies, mind and spirit. You are merely providing the vehicle for them to heal with your intentions and your magnetic applications.

Some will experience immediately and continued release from discomfort and pain while other more complex issues can take months to remedy, it all depends on the individual and their issues.

Biomagnetism session is a learning and healing session. During the first few minutes an interview is conducted to understand the reasons behind the health visit. Pairs of lightweight medium intensity magnets are gently placed on your body over your clothing, targeting Biomagnetic Pairs whose pH levels are imbalanced or on a surrogate if facilitating healing at a distance. Magnets remain on the soul for a determined amount of time-based on the geographic latitude of where the therapy is being conducted. After a healing session, one may experience a Herxheimer effect. The Herxheimer Reaction is a short-term (from days to a few weeks) detoxification reaction in the body. As the body detoxifies, it is not uncommon to experience flu-like symptoms including headache, joint and muscle pain, body aches, sore throat, general malaise, sweating, chills, nausea or other symptoms. In a die-off reaction, there is a release of toxins, proteins, and oxidizing agents that can result in an increase in inflammatory cytokines such as tumor necrosis factor alpha, interleukin-6, and interleukin-8.These symptoms can include: fatigue, brain-fog, muscle and nerve pain, chills and sweats, and/or memory and thinking.

Dr. Garcia has greatly reduced resulting Herxhemier type reactions after a healing session by conducting reservoir placements after each session work as called for. This further breaks up the toxic pathogens into bite size bytes and bits that then can be used as fuel for food the healthy cells to grow again and not need to be extricated out the body.

Personally, my role to heal another is as a "Facilitator". Not someone who is 'fixing' or 'making better' the soul rather I am facilitating their own Self-healing as they can learn for themselves the magnet placements to continue to heal themselves. Being a 'facilitator' also gets by the Medical mafia police since they souls are healing themselves, you are merely assisting their healing.

I then will follow the Beyond Biomag Scan Protocols of Dr. Garcia's, followed by issues and symptoms excel spreadsheet, then emotional scans for physical issues.

After I have finished, usually between ½ hour to 1-hour time, I muscle test and ask if the soul needs a follow up? And/or if they need to do magnet placements themselves to help with their healing. (Sidebar: always good to have extra magnets to give out, or they will want to take yours.☺)

Intentional Remote Healing aka Spooky Healing at a Distance

~ National Library of Medicine (NCBI) titled, *Distant Healing Intention Therapies: An Overview of the Scientific Evidence.*

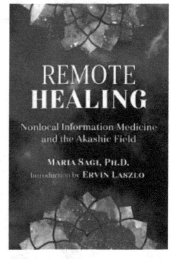

"In 2008 and 2009, the Cochrane Collaboration reported 2 systematic reviews, the first examining non-contact TT, healing touch, and Reiki and the second intercessory prayer. From the Reiki review, out of 24 randomized controlled trials (RCTs), a total of 1153 participants exposed to TT **had significantly lower average pain intensity** than unexposed participants, and trials conducted by more experienced practitioners appeared to yield greater effects. Larger effects were also found in Reiki studies in trials conducted by more experienced practitioners. By contrast, the intercessory prayer review did not demonstrate therapeutic efficacy. Out of 10 RCTs involving 7646 patients, there was no overall effect of intercessory prayer on prolonging life, general clinical state, readmission to coronary care unit, or rehospitalization.

Today, the "nonlocal", remote healing at a distance connections of quantum entanglement have been convincingly demonstrated. Throughout history and in virtually all cultures, reports can be found of individuals who could purportedly heal solely through their caring intentions. Today, the ancient shamanic tradition of healing — or harming — through the application of focused intentions is still vibrantly alive.[2] We refer to these practices generically as "**distant healing intention**" (DHI) therapies. The present article does not provide a systematic or exhaustive review of the relevant literature. Rather, we have selected representative portions to provide a high level overview of scientific studies of DHI".

This study, among several others validate remote distance healing can be done and proven, yet prayer was not recorded as being as significant in healing in this study.

Most know of the work of Dr. Emoto with intention and water crystals. In 1994, he conducted several experiments in which his team of researchers observed the effects of spoken word, prayer, music, and images on crystals of frozen water. The photographs captured in response to these stimuli revealed "beautiful crystals" forming in response to positive words and phrases, music, and "pure prayer." Conversely, when spoken to

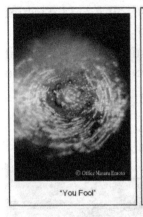
"You Fool"

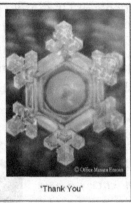
"Thank You"

or influenced negatively, the water molecules appeared disfigured and broken in the photographs (Emoto, 2010). Dr. Emoto chose to focus his research on water molecules because water comprises approximately 70% of the fluids in the human body, so the connection is obvious. For years, Dr. Emoto has been publishing the results of his studies in his *Messages from Water* book series. He was even to effect change at a distance having a non-local set intentions with success on the frozen crystalized water.

As Dr. Garcia has stated many times, "Biomag Healing is in its very, very infancy of development". When I asked him what his goal was overall for Biomag Healing he simply stated, "Nothing less than to heal the world!". Through his dedicated work and his willingness to share his knowledge with non-medical and medical communities, we are at the very beginning of realizing his dream and noble intentions.

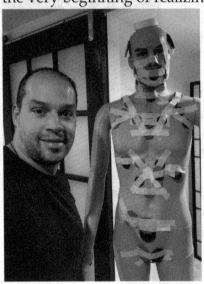

As I began to apply Dr. Garcia's healing protocols using a live surrogate for remote healing it became problematic in getting a live person to lay on the massage table to work with and through to remotely help another soul, who, likely, I have never met or never knew. The unified force *knows* how to find the intended soul you wish to conduct the healing protocols.

It became problematic for me to find live surrogates to come to my country home to conduct sessions through. On one occasion, a soul in great suffering needed my help as I had promised. Unfortunately, the surrogate cancelled, and I had no live person to work with, so I improvised and put several placements on a buddha statue in my home with my intention to help this soul remotely. When I informed Dr. Garcia what I had done he replied, "Oh sure, I sometimes, when I have no one to help, I will use a white board with a human image and place magnets, with my intention to help remotely"..he then added, "..it's all about the intention".

Thus I began a trial and experiment with using a mannequin to conduct healing remote sessions and right from the start instead of alive assistant and was amazed to find months on now that I am getting the same results as if I was using a live surrogate!

(However, having someone to work with is preferable in that you can ask questions as issues arise as well as they recalling issues sparked by your scan findings.)

I then began to think about if I could affix magnets of over 300 of Dr. Garcia's placements from his bible book, it would greatly decrease time and also dial in the putting the magnetic pairs correctly on the body and permanently without using rolls of masking tape. It worked! It works!

Whereas, Dr. Goiz's original healing protocol would take up to 4 hours to scan with one magnet placement, check the feet, do another, check the feet,…over 200 times each session was laborious and time consuming. With Dr. Garcia's scan sheets pairs can be placed at a time, greatly reducing overall time yet he still must get out of his chair for each placement.

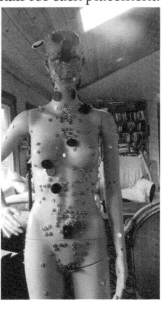

However remotely, and using finger scanning, we can set our intention, if the magnet pairs are already set on the **Maggyquin** and go onto the next placement thereby saving critical time and being able to scan more in the time allowed. This has greatly reduced the scan and healing sessions well under 1 hr. in most soul sessions. With the hundreds of placements to scan for, we now only need to set our intention to activate a common placement pair and only add magnets for more power as needed.

Now, anyone can use an inanimate surrogate, a doll, a wired human figure, or even a 2-dimensional stick figure. We are now playing with magnetic paint to see if we can have a surrogate that we can have open to place magnets at will, and easily.

Imagine if everyone had a magnetic laced Manny or Maggy Quin in their homes and literally can set their intention, with

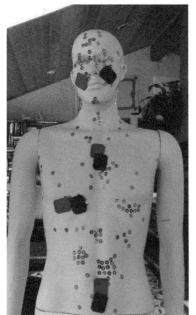

knowledge of placements needed and heal one another?

Another option is to paint the Maggy or Manny Quin with magnetic paint. I used two coats of paint and the smaller magnets stick beautifully. I then coded each placement from Dr. Garcia's Practioners Guide pages to the doll where the placements go. Now, all I have to do is look up the number in the book for a placement and put the magnets needed directly to the doll in the specified areas. Again, saving time, energy, tape as well as doing placements in the correct spots over and over again.

You can also number and personal pair placements, Most Common Pathogens, emotional placements and much, much more and saves valuable time during remote session work. Is remote healing as effective as hands on placements of magnets with a soul, in my opinion it is a resounding "ABSOLUTELY".

However, having said that, when you are with the soul you can find more issues, bring up more subjects and ask them about issues you might now find when doing remote scanning and placements. They also can learn more about Biomag Healing so it's a win/win for all, but either method works.

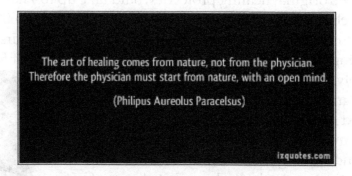

The art of healing comes from nature, not from the physician.
Therefore the physician must start from nature, with an open mind.

(Philipus Aureolus Paracelsus)

izquotes.com

Chapter 4

Principles of Healing with Magnets

What are Magnets. Types of Rare Earth Magnets. Magnets in Everyday Life. Remote Healing at a Distance with Magnets. Subtle Vibrational Healing Energy. Remote Viewing. Next Level of Biomag Healing ~ Spiritual Cleansing.

What Are Magnets?

Any object that exhibits magnetic properties is called a magnet. Every magnet has two points, or poles, where most of its strength is concentrated; these are designated as a north-seeking pole, or north pole, and a south-seeking pole, or south pole, because a suspended magnet tends to orient itself along a north-south line. Since a magnet has two poles, it is sometimes called a magnetic dipole, being analogous to an electric dipole, composed of two opposite charges. The like poles of different magnets repel each other, and the unlike poles attract each other.

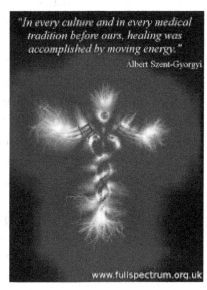

"In every culture and in every medical tradition before ours, healing was accomplished by moving energy."
Albert Szent-Gyorgyi

www.fullspectrum.org.uk

One remarkable property of magnets is that whenever a magnet is broken, a north pole will appear at one of the broken faces and a south pole at the other, such that each piece has its own north and south poles. It is impossible to isolate a single magnetic pole, regardless of how many times a magnet is broken or how small the fragments become. (The theoretical question as to the possible existence in any state of a single magnetic pole, called a monopole, is still considered open by physicists; experiments to date have failed to detect one.)

From his study of magnetism, C. A. Coulomb in the 18th century found that the magnetic forces between two poles followed an inverse-square law of the same form as that describing the forces between electric charges. The law states that the force of attraction or repulsion between two magnetic poles is directly proportional to the product of the strengths of the poles and inversely proportional to the square of the distance between them.

As with electric charges, the effect of this magnetic force acting at a distance is expressed in terms of a field of force. A magnetic pole sets up a field in the space around it that exerts a force on magnetic materials. The field can be visualized in terms of lines of induction (similar to the lines of force of an electric field). These imaginary lines indicate the direction of the field in a given region. By convention they originate at the north pole of a magnet and form loops that end at the south pole either of the same magnet or of some other nearby magnet (see also flux, magnetic). The lines are spaced so that the number per unit area is proportional to the field strength in a given area. Thus, the lines converge near the poles, where the field is strong, and spread out as their distance from the poles increases.

The Biomagnetic Pair of Opposites Attracting

The Biomagnetic Pair is defined as the set of charges that identify a pathology and that are constituted by two charges of opposite polarity. They are formed at the expense of the fundamental alteration of the pH of the organs that support it and are in vibrational and energetic resonance. The NEL defines the bioenergetic limits where all the cellular metabolic processes are carried out under the normal conditions of temperature (between 96.8o and 98.7oF), electromagnetic absorption (in the order of 400 to 700 nm) and pH (in the range of 7 +/- 0.3).

The bioenergetic alteration of the NEL obeys the "Law of All or Nothing", referring to when a phenomenon takes an organ out of its NEL and it persists regardless of whether the phenomenon which caused it continues to persist or not. It also seems that said energy limit is in the order of 1000 Gauss, since the bioenergetic depolarization, by means of natural magnets, also obeys charges over 1000 Gauss. Because of this, we must consider the normal manifestations of living organisms to be within the NEL, and pathological manifestations to exist outside of it.

Types of Rare Earth Magnets

It is first critical to understand the difference between the male principle of force, **EL**ectricity and the female law of attraction, **MAG**netism. Electricity is not created, it is 'managed' and 'transferred'. It can be 'stepped up' or 'stepped down' but now created.

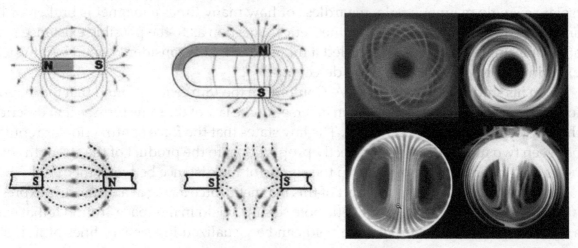

Magnetism has 3 main principle forces. Diamagnetism, Paramagnetism and Ferromagnetism. It CREATES energy through attraction and repulsion and eternal, omnipresent force in the Aether that Nikola Tesla was said to have tapped into to create free energy by grounding a rod into earth and running a conducting antenna into the sky above. That was over 100 years ago and we still don't have free energy for all.

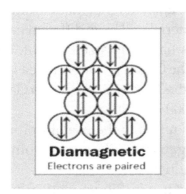

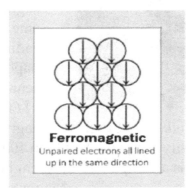

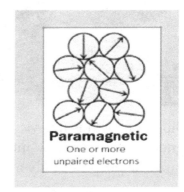

1) **Ferromagnetism** occurs when the magnetic moments in a magnetic material line up spontaneously at a temperature below the so-called Curie temperature, to produce net magnetization. The magnetic moments are aligned at **random** at temperatures above the Curie point, but become ordered, typically in a vertical or, in special cases, in a spiral (heliacal) array, below this temperature.

2) **Paramagnetism** is a weak form of magnetism observed in substances which display a positive response to an applied magnetic field. This response is described by its magnetic susceptibility per unit volume, which is a dimensionless quantity defined by the ratio of the magnetic moment to the magnetic field intensity. Paramagnetism is observed, for example, in atoms and molecules with an odd number of electrons, since here the net magnetic moment cannot be zero.

3) **Diamagnetism** is associated with materials that have a negative magnetic susceptibility. It occurs in nonmagnetic substances like graphite, copper, silver and gold, and in the superconducting state of certain elemental and compound metals. The negative magnetic susceptibility in these materials is the result of a current induced in the electron orbits of the atoms by the applied magnetic field. The electron current then induces a magnetic moment of opposite sign to that of the applied field. The net result of these interactions is that the material is shielded from penetration by the applied magnetic field.

It is easiest for me to think of Diamagnetism is the repulsion forces when two like polarities (- -, or + +) are facing one another. Paramagnetism are two forces attracting one another north and south. Ferromagnetism is the Aether, the Earth's toroidal field, the omnipresent energy in Mother Earth and Father Sky.

Jumping Jack Flash, It's About the Gauss

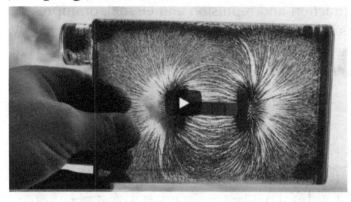

The Gauss of a magnet refers to the magnetic strength properties of a specific magnetic material which is used to compare and rate different magnets. Each magnet made from the same material will have different gauss readings based on size, weight, and shape. The Gauss is a subset measurement of the Telsa which where a Gauss is 1/10,000 of a Tesla.

(Biomagnetism is not *Magnetotherapy*. Single use magnets refers to the use of unipolar magnetic fields from low-intensity magnets (less than 1000 gauss) used for symptomatic therapeutic purposes only and is a completely different healing protocol).

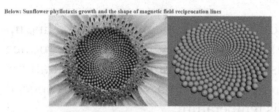

Below: Sunflower phyllotaxis growth and the shape of magnetic field reciprocation lines

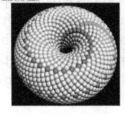
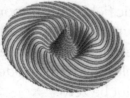

Below: Left, torus centrifugal flow around a disk magnet, right magnetic pressure gradients with high pressures showing raised, not to scale. This same pattern on the right is reproduced in electrification of the dielectric inertial plane against a magnetic field over time.

Magnets for use in Biomagnetism must have at least 1,000 surface Gauss so that they may provide the proper benefit. Magnets are usually rated in terms of the Core Gauss or the Maximum magnetic force at the dead center of a magnet. This is usually almost 10 times stronger than the surface gauss.

Therefore, a magnet with 1,500 surface gauss will have about 14,000 core Gauss. In order for Biomagnetism to function correctly, magnets of at least 1,000 surface gauss or 11,000 Core gauss or BrMax gauss or N40 or above ratings are desired for optimal use.

Using and applying these magnets in the proper locations found in Dr. Garcia's **Beyond Biomag 3D app (usbiomag.com) and** his Biomag Practioners Guide may help sustain normal metabolism in our bodies. Give some of these pairs a try and observe how you feel afterward. On the Beyond Biomag 3D ap you can use the dictionary search function in the app to identify the proper magnet pair placements and address the desired health interpretations.

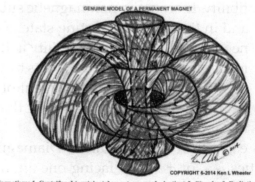

GENUINE MODEL OF A PERMANENT MAGNET

COPYRIGHT 6-2014 Ken L Wheeler

Magnetism: 1. Centrifugal (centripetal on return = polarization) 2. Circular 3. Radiative 4. Spatial
Dielectricity: 1. Centripetal 2. Radial 3. Inertial 4. Counterspatial

"Superlight" Magnetism

Engineer and Researcher, Dr. John Milewski is "part wizard, part mad scientist". An internationally-recognized leader and consultant in the field of advanced materials, Dr. John Milewski is a scientist, inventor, entrepreneur, writer, publisher, editor, and lecturer. He is primarily known for his work with magnetite and his protocols for magnetizing water. Over the last few decades, SuperLight aka Magnetricirty, has become a core concern of his research. Dr. John Milewski describes Magnetricity (known to mystics and metaphysicians as the nous, chi, and orgone or zero point energy) as the opposite of electromagnetic energy, revealing the previously unacknowledged parity of light. Instead of traveling away from a source at light speed, Magnetism is emitted from black holes and travels towards the source some ***10 billion times faster than the speed of light!***

Mathematically, magnetic energy travels at the speed of light squared to the 10th power! It has a frequency 10 billion times higher and has a corresponding and shorter wavelength than electricity. *It therefore has a higher energy density.* The question one asks immediately is, "If magnets are so powerful, how come we do not feel it, or how come it is not detected scientifically?" Well, the frequency is so high, its wave length so short, (4×10^{-8} nano–meters, or 4×10^{-17} meters), its velocity so fast, that it goes through everything as though the substance was nearly completely transparent (like glass). We can say the higher frequency is completely penetrating like x–rays, but even more so. Magnetricity is the unseen force in nature that has been ignored by science but real to the mystics and metaphysicians for thousands of years.

It has been given different names by different cultures for thousands of years such as Prana, Chi, Biomagnetic Energy, Wilhelm Reich's Orgone Energy, Tesla's Free Earth Energy, Animal Magnetism, Space Energy, Vacuum Energy, and Zero Point Energy, etc. Those who have subtle perception know it is real. Magnetism was identified scientifically over 100 years ago when James Clerk Maxwell solved his famous wave equation. This occurred shortly after radio was re-invented by Nikola Tesla, and theoretical physicists tried to find a mathematical model to explain radio waves. When using positive numbers in Maxwell's Equations this explains radio waves and also all forms of electro–magnetic radiation such as light, radio, TV, microwaves, x–rays, etc. What his equation also explains 100 years ago was Magnetricity but because it was the solution that comes from the use of negative numbers, "this second solution" was ignored for over 100 years.

Magnetiricity, some call the "Aether", is the prime activating energy in the universe and accounts for the production of what we call life. Aetheric magnetic energy interacts with special forms of matter in our bodies and produces what we call Vital Life Forces. These special forms of matter are found in bones, microcrystals and in the various fluids in the body, that contain cell salts. There are also, believed to be organic molecules in some body fluids, that are believed to be liquid crystalline in structure. These change state (liquid to crystal) very readily, with an extremely small change in energy (e.g. emotions). It is then no coincidence that when we muscle test using our brainwaves to ask questions, the response is immediate and imperceptible as to time between the question posed and the muscles response. As you can see from the chart, our brains have hundreds of millions of tiny magnetite crystals in our brain alone!

Proof of magnetic antennas in the brain

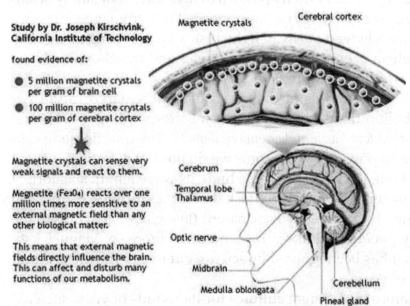

Study by Dr. Joseph Kirschvink, California Institute of Technology

found evidence of:

● 5 million magnetite crystals per gram of brain cell

● 100 million magnetite crystals per gram of cerebral cortex

Magnetite crystals can sense very weak signals and react to them.

Magnetite (Fe₃O₄) reacts over one million times more sensitive to an external magnetic field than any other biological matter.

This means that external magnetic fields directly influence the brain. This can affect and disturb many functions of our metabolism.

Magnetite crystals · Cerebral cortex · Cerebrum · Temporal lobe · Thalamus · Optic nerve · Midbrain · Medulla oblongata · Pineal gland · Cerebellum

In a human brain there are tens of billions of neurons, and they are of several sorts. Each neuron is equipped with approximately a thousand synapses, which are junction sites connecting the cells to each other. *Each synapse has ten million or so receptors. The number of neurons is frequently estimated at ten billion.* If one stretches out the DNA contained in the nucleus of a human cell, one obtains a two-yard-long thread that is only ten atoms wide. This thread is a billion times longer than its own width. Relatively speaking, it is as if your little finger stretched from Paris to Los Angeles. A thread of DNA is much smaller than the visible light humans perceive. Even the most powerful optical microscopes cannot reveal it, because DNA is approximately 120 times narrower than the smallest wavelength of visible light. The DNA molecule is a single long chain made up of two interwoven ribbons that are connected by the four bases. These bases can only match up in specific pairs—A with T, G with C. Any other pairing of the bases is impossible, because of the arrangement of their individual atoms: A can bond only with T, G only with C. This means that one of the two ribbons is the back-to-front duplicate of the other and that the genetic text is double: It contains a main text on one of the ribbons, which is read in a precise direction by the transcription enzymes, and a backup text, which is inverted and most often not read.

The original pairs of DNA were two females! They were *'attracted'* to one another. They then created two male to pair bond with. From these two pairs of DNA a replication is made, called RNA. Bottom line is that the Femine Devine IS the Creator being between male and female from the very DNA of all our existences! At the beginning of all DNA creation are two female DNA's that then create two male partners and then the two pairs create the RNA replicant. RNA is the operating system that body calls on to repair itself since it hosts the original operating instructions of our bodies in its base form.

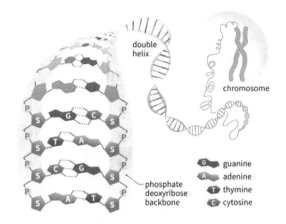

Magnetic Mind and Earth

"Whatever the repercussions, we have no alternative but to take seriously the possibility that Man has a magnetic sense of direction. Our body is electronic in nature and it is composed of millions and billions of micro–electronic units that are formed in structures that have a phase array organization. I believe that the electronic resonance in these organized conductive molecules, have some resonance with very small amounts of magnetic energies and that these energy fields and currents are responsible for the human aura and the energy vortexes found in the body chakra area. They also produce the Vital Life Forces in Nature". Robin Baker

In the 1980s, Robin Baker from the University of Manchester carried out a series of experiments to show that humans could sense magnetic fields. He took busloads of blind-folded volunteers on winding journeys for several kilometres before asking them to point their way back home. They did so more often than expected, and if they wore magnets on their heads, their accuracy dropped. The results were published in *Science* and you can read Baker's own description of his study in this 1980 issue of New Scientist. He even wrote a book about it. Since magnets are so powerful, even a very, very small amount produces more than enough energy to sustain life. Thus, life is produced and sustained by specific forms and amounts of organized matter, and old age

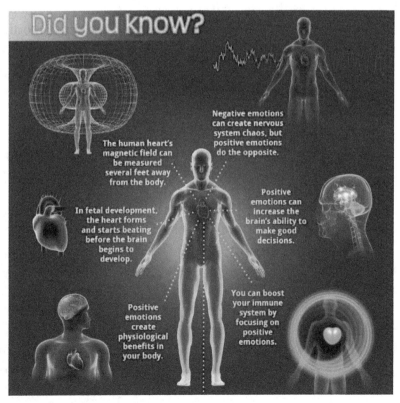

and eventual death occurs when too much disorder and disease comes into our bodies and breaks up this ordered structure.

At that point, the body can no longer produce enough Vital Life Force from magnetic energies to sustain itself. All forms of organized matter produce its own aura–finger–prints or energy signature when it reacts with our energy magnetic fields".

Vital Subtle Energy ~ Magnetricity not Electromagnetism

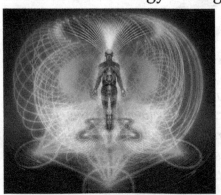

The modern Biofield viewpoint that is emerging has striking parallels in ancient viewpoints such as the Tibetan, Vedic and Jain medical traditions, where concepts of energy and information patterns are fundamental.

For example:

Jain teachings describe the interaction of the soul's consciousness with the karmic field, producing emanations known as *adhyavasāya* which interact with a subtle body called the *tejas sarir* ("fiery body") which supports mental and physical health, and are described in a manner resembling modern descriptions of magnetrical fields. Similarly, the Vedic concept of the energetic body known as *prānamayakoṣa*, and the Tibetan Buddhist description of a subtle body known as the "*vajra body*" (Sanskrit:*vajradeha*; Tibetan: *sku rdorje* or *rdo rje lus*) refer to a network of invisible energy channels that guide bodily functions.

Energy healing has 2 main principles:

- The presence of God is within everyone. Certainly, this presence has the resources necessary to affect any healing. It is fine if you don't believe in God, because a disbelief in God will not stop the healing– everyone and everything contains the organizing intelligence of the whole creation.

- What we think of as "our body" is actually a continuum of intelligence. It spans the quantum level of creation that underlies its cells to the densest level of creation, our physical reality.

Presence of God/Divine Intelligence

The universe exists in layers. There is a non-changing, eternal level of God which is beyond all exists in time and space. And there is also a level of this Divine Intelligence residing within each of us. That level changes as we change. And it evolves as we evolve.

A beautiful web of life connects all parts of creation to each other. This living matrix of filaments also spans all dimensions of space and time. Distance Energy Work occurs through this communication network. It allows us to heal the past–the existence of the web of life allows the past and future to collapse into the eternally present moment.

Muscle scanning connects us to this Divine Intelligence to help direct and guide us to the appropriate magnet placements for healing.

What is Energy Healing: The Four Denser Bodies

The four denser or lower bodies are usually associated with the present life and are more manifest, apparent and familiar to us.

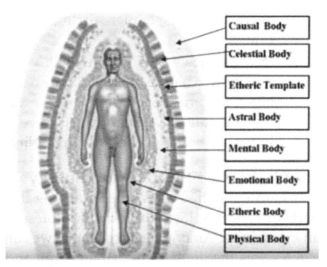

1. **Physical body** – We are most familiar with our physical body, comprised of organs and organ systems. Imbalances are sometimes sitting at very fine levels of this layer. In order to eliminate these imbalances, our vision must travel like a microscope to the deepest levels of the physiology.

2. **Aetheric Body** – The aetheric body is an energetic map of the physical form. It looks like the physical body but not as dense. Often the experience of physical pain is held in this body. For instance, it is possible to feel pain in a limb or organ that is physically missing.

3. **Mental Body** – The mental body comprises conscious mind, subconscious mind, unconscious mind and the avenue of awareness. We create certain role-playing games from this level of being.

4. **Emotional Body** – The emotional body is the body of desire, and this is also the body of feelings. Our "gut feelings" originate from here. Intuition arises as an integration between the mental and emotional bodies.

The Four Subtle Bodies

These layers associate with the permanent self and are multidimensional. They are closer to the unmanifest, eternal, absolute field of life.

1. **Astral Body** – The astral body is the densest level of the subtler bodies. It acts as shielding for the body. When healthy, its appearance is smooth, like fine filaments of light aligned together. When healthy, the astral body has a somewhat resilient texture that disallows the invasion of other energy forms such as viruses, intentions, thought forms, etc.

2. **Causal Body** – This level has seven rays or layers and contains mechanisms, or energy organs. These subtle organs direct Divine energy or intelligence into specific

channels to give rise to the more manifested levels of creation. All collective forms of self are here, including angels, devas, gods, as well as the realms of creation. At its finest level, the causal body takes on the form of locations, or fields. Furthermore, resources for healing are most often implemented from this level of the body.

3. **Dynamic Silence –** This level is purely unmanifest, but just at the edge of awareness of its own nature. Here the three-in-one dynamics of consciousness function to create the first tender stirring of life. In Sanskrit this level is known as Saguna Brahm.

4. **Pure Silence –** This is pure quality-less, unmanifest Being that folds completely into its own nature. It is an infinite ocean of silence, resting within itself. In the gap between Pure Silence and Dynamic Silence there is a most delicate movement, or transformation of Being. This is where all the resources required for healing emerge. In Sanskrit, this level is known as Nirguna Brahm.

Ka, Qi, Prana ~ Subtle Vital Energy

According to the beliefs in force among the ancient Egyptians, man was made up of 9 parts or concepts, levels of formation present since his birth and which remained even after his death. Among these concepts, we can point out the "KA" and the "BA".

KA - was the double - the vital energy and, as in life, needed to have its needs fully satisfied by the energy of offerings, such as fruit, bread, poultry and wine. His priests were in charge of these procedures, and there were rituals in which these ceremonies were performed. The KA needed an energetic support and, consequently, it would have a better result if it could find the conservation of the body, which was accomplished by mummification. Often, these objectives were also achieved by placing statues of the dead, placed in their own chapels - the SERDAB.BA - it was the soul or a dynamic concept, which could move, represented as a bird with a human head. This entity could visit the tomb, moving through the "false door". They considered it as a repository of the dead man's qualities - his soul - his divine essence. In sequence, it was the BA that answered the call of the priests, during the divine and funeral cults.

Prana [Sanskrit], in Ayurvedic tradition, is defined as the life force or vital energy that permeates the body and is especially concentrated along the midline in centers called the chakras. Pranayama is mentioned in verse 4.29 of the Bhagavad Gita, which has been dated to between the fifth and second century B.C.E.

Qi [Chinese] is defined as one of the most basic substances that, according to traditional Chinese medicine, pervades the body. It is a subtle influence or vital energy that is cause of most physiological processes and whose proper balance is necessary for maintaining health. Qi is also spelled chi, ch'i, and ki. The earliest representation of the Chinese character for qi is on a jade artifact dated from 481-221 B.C.E.

Our frequency of vibration depends on the amount of prana "life force energy" that is channeled through us emanating from Source.

Prana is the foundation and essence of all life; the energy and vitality that pervades the entire universe. It flows in everything that exists. It is the connection between the material world, consciousness and mind. Prana is distributed in the body through a network of the nadis "meridians" to every part of body. It is said there are 72,000 nadis in the human body. Among them are three important nadis:

Ida, the "Moon", connected with the left nostril

Pingala, the "Sun", connected with the right nostril

Sushumna, the "Central Nadi", within the spinal column.

Ida and pingala criss-cross each other at seven chakras along sushumna nadi creating energy vortexes. Each one is vibrating at a different frequency of vibration and is associated to an element. As we move up along sushumna nadi the elements become lighter and lighter, starting with the five physical elements of earth, water, fire, air, and ether, and then moving up through the spiritual elements of sound and light.

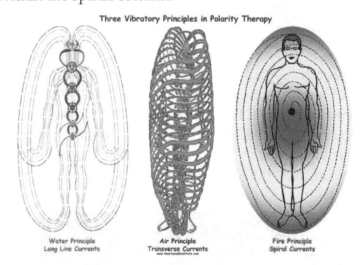

Three Vibratory Principles in Polarity Therapy

Water Principle
Long Line Currents

Air Principle
Transverse Currents
www.heartwoodinstitute.com

Fire Principle
Spiral Currents

The Serpent symbols also represent Free Energy (Spirit/Spiral) like when two copper coils are intertwined around a rare earth magnet you have just created a hermetic marriage of electromagnetic energy! The human body is powered by our kundalini, or Life Force. By placing two pillars with copper wires around powerful magnets you have created free energy called a "Torus Field". The Tesla Coil is based off of ancient Antiquitechnology, or Serpent Technology, passed down by the Nagas (serpent or dragon).

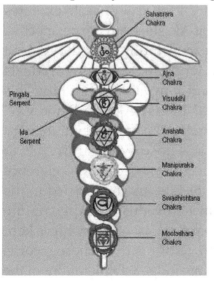

Sahasrara Chakra

Ajna Chakra

Pingala Serpent

Visuddhi Chakra

Ida Serpent

Anahata Chakra

Manipuraka Chakra

Swadhishtana Chakra

Mooladhara Chakra

Another claim is that the word magnet comes from the ancient Greeks. It is thought to derive from Magnes lithos, meaning "stone from Magnesia," an area of Greece that was known for its volcanic rocks with magnetic attributes. The Greek philosopher Aristotle spoke about using magnets as a healing therapy. In ancient Greece, Aristotle practice included magnets for healing purposes, and relieving pain. He was one of the first to document his findings in 111 B.C.

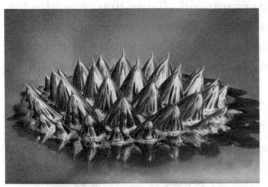

Magnetic energy fields in ferro fluid under light.

One of the earliest references to the Akashic Records in modern times was made by Helena Blavatsky, founder of the Theosophical movement in the late 19th century. Theosophy is an esoteric belief system that incorporates philosophical tenets from eastern religions while maintaining that "there is no religion higher than Truth."

Blavatsky claimed she learned of the records from Tibetan monks, or "mahatmas" who said the records could be found in the "akasha," or "akasa," the Sanskrit word for astral light, or the ether element in eastern belief systems. This fifth element of space is considered the fundamental fabric of reality from which all other elements emerge — the source of material reality. The eastern idea of karma is a major facet of the akashic records.

These "Masters of the Ancient Wisdom," as Blavatsky referred to them as, taught her clairvoyance, psychic abilities, and astral projection. She used these tools to channel information from the akashic records and built a large following of Theosophists, including some famous ones.

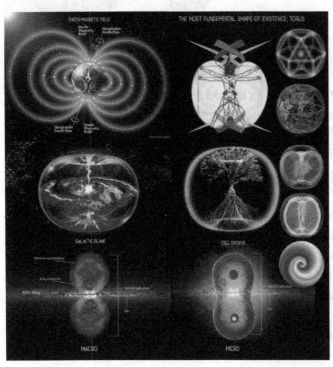

Metaphysician Rudolf Steiner also referenced the Akashic Records, asserting that every action, word, and thought leaves a trace in etheric realms. Contemporary physicist Ervin Laszlo explores concepts of Akasha from the perspective of science, concluding that the Akasha contains templates for human ideals such as harmony and equanimity. This is reflected in his "Akasha Paradigm" which he relates to human evolutionary processes. Those who subscribe to Akashic record models often reference the Book of Life first mentioned in the old testament (Exodus). Biblical scripture asserts that a record of every life is kept in heaven, and it is from these records that souls are judged. Explorations of the akashic field were also a major focus of the writings and work of Edgar Cayce. Cayce's Akashic studies posited that there is a storehouse of information in a non-physical plane of existence, which maintains a record of every soul's past, present, and future. Cayce's readings are some of the best known.

In the Akasha, every thought, idea, and action from the past, present, and future is stored ad infinitum. If you're familiar with String Theory, the Akashic Records is basically like a database of what's happening in all the universes that are co-existing together. The Akashic Records are basically a record of what will happen, is happening, or has happened. Because they are a higher dimension, the rules of time don't really apply. Time is a FLAT circle to the Akashic Records, so information from 2,000 years ago is as accessible as what happened to you yesterday. And what happened to you yesterday is as available as what could happen to you — if you stay on the same destiny trajectory — in 10 years.

CIA Remote Viewing and Targeting

The movie, "Men Who Stare Out Goats" was a very poor rendition of the Stargate Project conducted by General Albert Stubblebine as described here by Wikipedia:

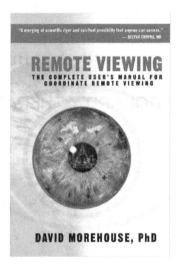

Stargate **Project** was the 1991 **code name** for a secret **U.S. Army** unit established in 1978 at **Fort Meade, Maryland,** by the **Defense Intelligence Agency** (DIA) and **SRI International** (a California contractor) to investigate the potential for **psychic** phenomena in military and domestic intelligence applications. The Project, and its precursors and sister projects, originally went by various code names — *GONDOLA WISH, GRILL FLAME, CENTER LANE, PROJECT CF, SUN STREAK, SCANATE* — until 1991 when they were consolidated and rechristened as "Stargate Project".

Stargate Project work primarily involved **remote viewing,** the purported ability to psychically "see" events, sites, or **information** from a great distance. [1] The project was overseen until 1987 by Lt. Frederick Holmes "Skip" Atwater, an aide and "psychic headhunter" to Maj. Gen. **Albert Stubblebine**, and later president of the **Monroe Institute**.[2] The unit was small-scale, comprising about 15 to 20 individuals, and was run out of "an old, leaky wooden barracks".[3]

The Stargate Project was terminated and declassified in 1995 after a **CIA** report concluded that it was never useful in any intelligence operation. Information provided by the program was vague and included irrelevant and erroneous data.

The project went underground when information about the program was leaked. It was highly successful, as validated by the many books and those who worked on the projects, including civilian Stephen Schwarz, Ingo Swan and many others who wrote extensively about the projects they worked on.

In 2009, I attended a weekend workshop hosted by Mr. Stephen Schwarz at the Esalen Institute on the Pacific Coast of mid-California. There I learned, was shown and proved to myself, the abilities we all have to access the Akashic Record of all things known and unknown, like the military had done for decades with millions of research to spend. I was able to detect issues and symptoms in the person next to me as well as describe, abstractly, an image yet to be presented on the screen to the class by Mr. Schwarz. Mr. Schwarz told the story of two remote viewers who were placed 1500 ft. underwater in a submarine down off the Catalina Islands near San Diego, California. Two 'targets' were identified located somewhere in Northern California, and the remote viewers were able to get first class "hits" or identifications abstractly on the whereabouts and surroundings of the two targets they were trying to locate. The experiment was to see if remote viewing could be conducted underwater successfully and was proven successful. (Remote viewing deals with abstract object viewing and interpreters determine location, object, etc).

Next Level Biomagnetic Healing ~
Clearing Body, Mind, Soul and Spirit

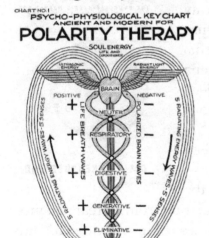

Depending on the individual soul I am intending to help and assist their healing, remotely or in person, my intention is always to achieve optimal well-being.

I think of my session work with the individual as diagnosing and doing placements on a tree of the soul I am wishing to help facilitate their healing.

I begin with the low hanging fruit of the issues (i.e. pain, insomnia, fatigue, chronic ailments, etc.). Dr. Garcia's Bible lists over 300 placements for physical issues. Next, I focus on the emotions and mental state of the soul or the branches and the trunk of the issues. This is usually my 2nd or 3rd session, if needed.

I ask the body to respond to any emotional or mental issues that are affecting their physical issues. Once I get the emotional response I drill down to the associated part of the body where placement pairs need to go. I then discuss with the soul about these emotions and ask if this soul needs to do some work to let go of the emotions causing the physical ailments, whether it be mediation, forgiveness, confront the issue, etc. Remember that 80% + of our physical issues are emotionally caused and driven, so dealing with the emotions can/will help physical recovery. Finally, I will ask if Spiritual clearing is also needed. The roots of many of our generational issues.

Spiritual Science of Clearing Demonic Energies

Luciferic are emotional issues and Ahrimanic are physical in nature and then there is the Azuric entities that will come forth in the near and distant future as Spiritual healing grows from its infancy stage today.

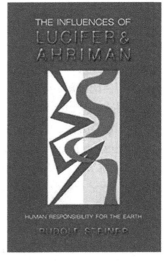

The final clearing and cleansing is getting to the **roots** of the issues to find homeostasis and optimal health in the Spiritual cleansing and purification of the soul I am assisting.

We are Mind, Body *and Soul.* As you read earlier by the likes of Rudolph Steiner and many others, Spiritual Science is destined to become part of our complete healing protocols in the 21st century.

Caution and care must be applied when using these techniques as we are dealing with Spirit bodies that can translocate if not transformed whereby the issues and ailments are simply transferred to another part of the body or to another being. Dr. Are Thoreson is one of foremost experts on Spiritual Clearing today.

Dr. Are Thoresen was born in Norway in 1952. A doctor of veterinary medicine, he has also studied anthroposophic medicine, homeopathy, acupuncture, osteopathy and agriculture. Since 1981 he has run a private holistic practice in Sandefjord, Norway, for the healing of small animals and horses, as well as people. He has lectured widely, specializing in veterinary acupuncture, and has published dozens of scholarly articles. In 1984 he started to treat cancer patients, both human and animals, and this work has been the focus of much of his recent research. He brings an anthroposophical approach to his healing of animals and humans over the past decades.

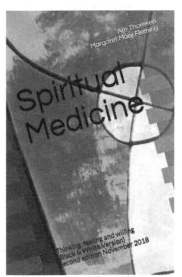

Dr. Thorsen points out that this work is about transforming the demonic energies rather than just translocating the energy which will just go to another host, possibly a partner or pet, or come back around in some other illness or symptom or ailment.

Ahrimanic influences are physical and Luciferian influences exist in the emotional and mental planes. When scanning you may ask which entity you are dealing with.

"All our diseases are caused by or effectuated by the cooperation of Ahrimanic ("The Double") and Luciferic Demons inhabiting our bodies. In most diseases there is a certain and individual distance between the two kinds of Demons. The stronger and less diseased the specific person or patient is the further the two types of Demons are parted. In healthy, young persons they may be 20 cm apart, in healthy horses 80 cm. In cancer the cooperation of these Demons is quite special, as they have joined closely together; there is almost no distance between them.

This lack of distance between the Ahrimanic and the Luciferic Demons makes it very difficult to heal as they have joined forces. It is much easier for them to stay put or if they have to translocate this is also quite problems for them. This is the curse of our present times, resulting in the explosion of cancer that we see rising in all countries of the world.

Then times that we are living in make it easier for the Demons to unite in the way described, and as such promote the cooperation of Luciferic and Ahrimanic forces. Our very time-spirit or rather lack of time-spirit brings them closer together, closer than ever before.

So what is it in out modern mentality and Spiritual composition of the human soul of today that can make this happen, this enhanced "friendship" between Ahriman and Lucifer?

The love of our material possessions and the lack of humility and belief in the Spiritual world (opens to Ahriman), combined with greed and lust for money and hatred towards the Spiritual world (opens to Lucifer), thus allowing the close cooperation and entrance of both the adversaries.

This counts both for the civilization at large. Not necessarily for the single individuals. Since 1984, I have treated more than a 1000 patients suffering from all kinds of cancer, both animals and humans. The results have been especially good in mammary cancer (85%), also in melanosarcoma (80%). Results in lymphosarcoma and brain cancer have been moderately good (70%). However, my results in liver cancer and pancreatic cancer were mediocre; the healing rate being "only" 60% in the few patients I have treated.

As I started to "see" the disease-bringing Demons more and more with my Spiritual Eyes, I understood more and more the necessity of hindering the described Translocation.

This was done by and through the understanding of Christ, the Middle-Point and the importance of not fighting the adversaries directly, but to transform them in love, as described in my book "7-fold way to therapy".

a. The Demons will not transform. In ordinary diseases they were not strong enough to withstand the middle-point, but the joined Demons in cancer had the strength to do so.

b. My ability to "see" the Demons brought about a possibility for the strongest Demons, especially in diseases where the Luciferic and the Ahrimanic Demons have joind forces) to change or Translocate, as described in Quantum Physics (when an elemental particle is seen it changes radically).

c. That I accepted that certain people could be allowed to earn money on my method. That invited in Mammon, a very strong Ahrimanic Demon.

d. The effect stopped for my students because we are "entangled", also described in Quantum Physics. This entanglement was only to my personal students, not to the ones that I had never met.

e. It has to do with some changes in the world. The world has changed in a way that enables the strongest Demons to endure, not the weaker ones.

n Quantum Physics there are two important laws:

1. The law of "Uncertainty", proposed by Werner Heisenberg.
2. The law of "Entanglement".

When I started to "see" the Elementals (in physics called the Elementary particles), they changed and were able to avoid me. Further that I am "entangled" with most of my students, so that the same will happen to them.

I now understand that the Demons try to defend themselves, to survive as Demons, even if they actually want to be transformed. And why do they have to defend themselves? Is it because I started to become too strong or dangerous for them because of the new way of treating diseases together with my "new" connection to Christ? Or is it because I "saw" then with my Spiritual Eyes, and thus enabling them to escape? Or is it that the finishing of my 40.000 years old Karma had come to an end? Or is it that Mammon had been allowed to have a finger within this project? Or a combination of these factors.

Before I always treated either the excess or the deficiency. Then the Demons could just Translocate, it was not so "dangerous" for them. Then, when I realized this Translocation more and more, and started to treat the Middle-Point to change the Demons, to dissolve then into the light, then they tried to avoid my treatment. They tried to find ways of withstanding the treatment. In "normal" diseases the Demons cannot avoid the transforming treatment, but in cancer the close cooperation of the Luciferic and the Ahrimanic Demons lead to a greater strength of the two Demons and they are thus able to avoid the Transformation.

At this stage I find it important to emphasize that the effect of cancer treatment, when based on a Spiritual foundation, is not at all stable or expected to be stable. I have seen through my life that the effect varies with several factors, of which the most important are:

1. The geographical location of both the therapist and the patient.
2. The directions of the mountains, if they are situated east-west or north-south.
3. The rigidity of the Etheric body of the patient.
4. How much the patient has meditated.
5. The knowledge of the therapist, especially Spiritual knowledge of the Demonic causes of the disease.
6. The karma of both the therapist and the patient.
7. The karma or strength of the disease itself, that is of the Demon(s) causing the disease.
8. The love and empathy between the therapist and the patient.

Then something unexpected happened. By the help of destiny I lectured in New York upstate and was to treat the participants of the course. I decided to treat according to the anatomical midpoint, the Christ point. 25 participants lay at the floor on the evening of 5th of November 2016, and I needled them all at the individual midpoint between Lucifer and Ahriman. The needling took 20 minutes. Then I sat back to watch. The needle that was placed on the stomach between the Adversaries seemed to activate the area left of "free" Etheric force, not dominated by Ahriman or Lucifer. This area became activated, became rhythmic and oscillating. After some time the Ahrimanic demons became more light-filled and started to float up from all the participants and started to circle around and over the whole group. The circling became more and more luminous going upwards in a male-stream. In the Light the face of an Angel appeared ... or an Archangel. One of the participants saw Michael. I went into the middle of the whirl and felt divine.

The needling of the Middle point caused an oscilation in the Etheric body just between the Ahrimanic and the Luciferic pathological structures. This oscilation in the different patients started to make a sympathetic resonance between the different members of the group, and the resonance multiplied the strength of the treatment to a very high degree, so that the whole group was drawn into the effect of the treatment, even those where the Ahrimanic and the Luciferic Demons were tight bound together, as they are in cancer. What I could not have done in such patients was done through the whole group.

The effect in a group was totally different as when treating single individuals. This understanding struck me like a light from heaven. Of course, the cooperation of the Demons had made them strong, so strong that they could withstand the single individual patient and treatment. The power of the group they could not withstand. The cooperation of the good in every and each one of the patients was then able to transform the evil into the light.

This described effect was stronger in the dawn and the dusk, as Etheric forces always are stronger at these times. Patients lying east-west also felt a stronger effect than those lying north-south.

Another way is for the Ahrimanic forces in addition to individualize the treatment is to mechanize it to maintain control, as the machines are in their dominion.

This can be fought or counteracted by placing Christ in the middle of a group of human patients. The group therapy based on the Christ middle point therapy showed me that this might be the right way to go.

"Where two or three are gathered in my name, there I am right in their middle".

According to Rudolf Steiner we will be more and more fused with technology and this will be utilized by the adversaries to gain access and control over the whole of human evolution. By using the social element of group treatment combined with the absence of machines, using only one single needle in the most healthy point of the body, namely the Christ point, we can go forward in preventing the disastrous cooperation between Lucifer and Ahriman creating the epidemic wave of cancer we see today.

Further we can in this way turn the whole medical sphere towards the spiritual conception of the world. ~ Dr. Are Thoreson

Dr. Thoreson uses acupuncture needles to separate the demons, yet you can set your intention or even set your magnets for each entity. I then open my heart and clear my mind and THANK the Luciferic or Ahrimanic demon for showing me where the issues lie and that I can now effect healing. I see the demons as just trying to help us with our deeper issues and once we have located and dealt with them, we invite those demons back into our hearts, to LOVE. I do not see demons as the enemy but those wishing to bring out attention to the deepest issues of humanity.

You must be Spiritually grounded and aware of how Spiritual demons operate and protect yourself before doing this kind of healing though.

Luciferian Entities = Emotions
Ahrimanic Entities = Physical
Azuric Entities = Spiritual

N52 Neodymium Magnets to Heal

The penetration value is how deep into the tissue the magnetic effect penetrates. It is very simple – if there is a deep tissue condition, the magnet must be strong enough to penetrate the energy to stimulate the cells correctly. Remember that the effect of the magnets is an all or nothing scenario. The magnets are either 100% effective, or they do no harm = 0% effective. All Biomagnetic healing N52 Neodymium magnets are designed to specifically reach the required A-Z penetration values. Dr. Goiz and Dr. Garcia both say that N52 Neodymium magnets are the only ones that should be used for BiomagHealing with a minimum of 1,000 Gauss.

Dubbed "The World's Strongest Permanent Magnet", neodymium magnets are magnets made of neodymium. To put their strength into perspective, they can produce magnetic fields with up to 1.4 Telsa. Neodymium is a rare-earth element featuring the atomic number 60. It was discovered in 1885 by chemist Carl Auer von Welsbach. It wasn't until nearly a century later until neodymium magnets were invented. The unparalleled strength of neodymium magnets makes them an excellent choice for a variety of commercial applications, some of which include the following:

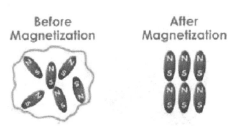

Before Magnetization   After Magnetization

Biomagnet Subtle Energy Polarity

Positive +	Negative -
Sun/Electricity	Moon/Magnet
Male/Apollo/Aries	Female/Isis/Venus
Pushing out	Pulling In
Creativity	Form
Repulsion	Attaction
Fire	Water
Entropy	Syntropy
Clockwise	Counterclockwise
Logical	Intuitive
Initiating	Nurturing

- Hard disk drives (HDDs) for computers
- Door locks
- Electric automotive engines
- Electric generators
- Voice coils
- Cordless power tools
- Power steering
- Speakers and headphones
- Retail decouplers

Modern technology would not exist without magnets! Rare earth magnets play a significant role in a wide range of devices including simple toys, computers, credit cards, MRI machines, and business equipment. Here are some examples.

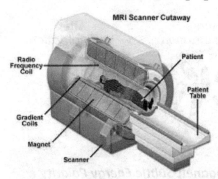

MRI Scanner Cutaway

Radio Frequency Coil
Patient
Patient Table
Gradient Coils
Magnet
Scanner

Health and Medicine Magnets are found in some commonly used medical equipment such as and Magnetic Resonance Imaging machines. MRIs use powerful magnetic fields to generate a radar-like radio signal from inside the body, using the signal to create a clear, detailed picture of bones, organs and other tissue. An MRI magnet is very strong – thousands of times more powerful than common kitchen magnets. Another medical use for magnets is for treating cancer. A doctor injects a magnetically-sensitive fluid into the cancer area and uses a powerful magnet to generate heat in the body. The heat kills the cancer cells without harming healthy organs.

Home Refrigerator magnets hold papers, bottle openers, and other small items to the metal refrigerator door. A pocket compass uses a magnetic needle to show which way is north. The dark magnetic strip on the backside of a credit card stores data in much the same way as a computer's hard drive does. Vacuum cleaners, blenders and washing machines all have electric motors that work by magnetic principles. You'll find magnets in phones, doorbells, shower curtain weights and children's toys.

Computers and Electronics Many computers use magnets to store data on hard drives. Magnets alter the direction of magnetic material on a hard disk in segments that then represent computer data. Later, computers read the direction of each segment of the magnetic material to "read" the data. The small speakers found in computers, televisions, and radios also use magnets; inside the speaker, a wire coil and magnet convert electronic signals into sound vibrations.

Maglev Trains Maglev Trains (derived from *magnetic levitation*) is a system of train transportation that uses two sets of magnets: one set to repel and push the train up off the track, and another set to move the elevated train ahead, taking advantage of the lack of friction. Along certain "medium-range" routes (usually 320 to 640 km [200 to 400 mi]), maglev can compete favorably with high-speed rail and airplanes.

With maglev technology, there is just one moving part: the train itself. The train travels along a guideway of magnets which control the train's stability and speed. Propulsion and levitation require no moving parts. Maglev vehicles have set several speed records and maglev trains can accelerate and decelerate much faster than conventional trains; The Shanghai maglev train, also known as the Shanghai Transrapid, has a top speed of 430 km/h (270 mph). The line is the fastest operational high-speed maglev train, designed to connect Shanghai Pudong International Airport and the outskirts of central Pudong, Shanghai. It covers a distance of 30.5 km (19 mi) in just over 8 minutes.

Magnetic "Earth Engine" Batteries and Free Clean Abundant Energy for All

Earth Engine is the world's first and only power source propelled by Asymmetrical Magnetic Propulsion. It can generate electricity, operate liquid pumps, air compressors, and other mechanical devices 24 hours a day, 365 days a year. It is fully independent of the power grid and offers significant cost savings over other technologies. Earth Engine creates constant, reliable, and renewable energy.

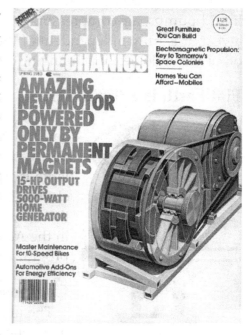

"What if I showed you a device that you could put in the back of a pickup and power a city block?" *says Inductance Energy Chief, Dennis M. Danzik.*

The generated power uses no fossil fuels, produces no heat, and requires no combustion. Earth Engine does not consume any fossil fuels, it does not run on the sun, the wind, hydro, bio-fuels, or radioactive fuel sources. It can run 24 hours a day, 7 days a week, 365 days a year creating constant energy unlike renewable technologies such as solar and wind. It is not reliant on a reaction or burning of fuel source. Earth Engine is the world's first and only power source propelled by Asymmetrical Magnetic Propulsion. It can generate electricity, operate liquid pumps, air compressors, and other mechanical devices 24 hours a day, 365 days a year. It is fully independent of the power grid and offers significant cost savings over other technologies. Earth Engine creates constant, reliable, and renewable energy. This is not a "theory". Inductance Energy is selling, and has installed these magnetic energy devices, in many locations in the United States to date, yet few know of their existence. Currently, IE has developed, manufactured,

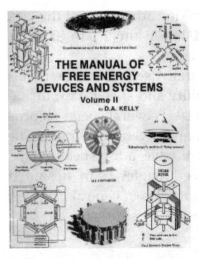

and is installing 7.5 to 25-kilowatt engines, capable of driving up to 4,000 pounds of inertia power and *delivering in excess of 25 kilowatts.*

Magnets in electric generators turn mechanical energy into electricity, while some motors use magnets to convert electricity back into mechanical work. In recycling, electrically powered magnets in cranes grab and move large pieces of metal, some weighing thousands of pounds. Mines use magnetic sorting machines to separate useful metallic ores from crushed rock. In food processing, magnets remove small metal bits from grains and other food. Farmers use magnets to catch pieces of metal that cows eat out in the field. The cow swallows the magnet with its food; as it moves through the animal's digestive system it traps metal fragments. It can generate electricity, operate liquid pumps, air compressors, and other mechanical devices 24 hours a day, 365 days a year. It is fully independent of the power grid and offers significant cost savings over other technologies. Earth Engine creates constant, reliable, and renewable energy.

Flat Earth is a Big Magnet!

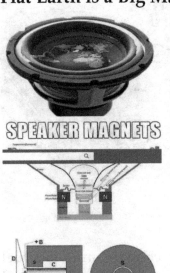

Earth is a big huge battery. The north pole is the negative polarity and the Antarctic Circle is the positive polarity surrounding Earth's land mass. It works just like a speaker works with a large magnet at the center. The salt in the ocean provides the electrolysis for alternating currents that produces free energy as the Tartarians proved and Telsa copied in his proof of free energy in the Aether at Wardenclyffe before J.P. Morgan defunded the program and burned it down.

Compasses and Navigation

The ancient Chinese are believed to have first used them in magnetic compasses for navigation purposes. They found out magnets could direct needles and correlated with the north pole and used that information to navigate. The early compasses have been created with lodestone because present-day magnets were no longer invented yet.

Lodestone comes from the mineral magnetite and is the handiest obviously occurring magnet. modern-day day magnets, like neodymium magnets and uncommon earth magnets, are crafted from a complicated process in which some of the metals are forged together. This technique helps to cause them to stronger and extra suitable for a way they're used today. Therefore, lodestone in comparison to sturdy uncommon earth magnets is weaker.

CERN Collider ~ A Massive Magnetic Earth Field

Is the CERN Large Hadron Collider in Switzerland being used to manipulate time? Is this why the how the Mandela effect is being caused by literally changing the historical records of time? There are also CERN Colliders being built around the world now. Note the imagery of CERN with the

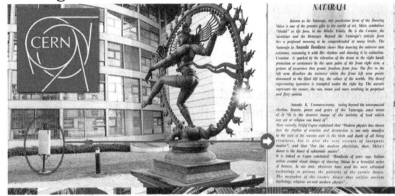

statue of Shiva, the Lord of Destruction as its symbol and the 666 Satanic symbolism in their logo as well. Why?

The permanent magnet is a long-time energy source. This has been shown for many years in the rating of magnets as **high** or **low** energy sources for many applications over long usage. The permanent magnet is the first room temperature super conductor. In fact, I believe that super conductors are simply large wound magnets. The current in a super conductor is not initiated by a strong emf, such as a battery, but is instead actually induced into existence by a magnetic field. Then, in order to determine how much current may be flowing in the super conductor coil, we measure its magnetic field. This appears to be something like going out the door and coming back in the window.

Another rather unique feature of super conductors is the fact that their magnetic lines of force experience a change in direction. No longer do these lines flow at right angles to the conductor, but they now exist parallel to the conductor. Theoretically, the heavy conductor currents exist in the fine filaments of niobium within each small wire of niobium

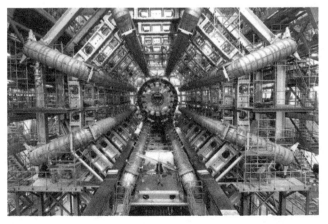

tin from which such super conductors are made. Isn't it interesting that the finer the wire the less the resistance until eventually there is no resistance at all?

The Massive CERN Collider runs on Magnets, we are told/sold, is to find the "God Particle", so they say. All the magnets on the LHC are electromagnets. The main dipoles generate powerful 8.3 tesla magnetic fields – more than 100,000 times more powerful than the Earth's magnetic field. The **electromagnets** use a current of 11,080 amperes to produce the field, and a superconducting coil allows the high currents to flow *without losing any energy to electrical resistance*. Thousands of "**lattice magnets**" on the LHC bend and tighten the particles' trajectory. They are responsible for keeping the beams stable and precisely aligned. **Dipole magnets**, one of the most complex parts of the LHC, are used to bend the paths of the particles. There are 1232 main dipoles, each 15 metres long and weighing in at 35 tons. If normal magnets were used in the 27 km-long LHC instead of superconducting magnets, the accelerator would have to be 120 kilometres long to reach the same energy. Powerful **magnetic fields** generated by the dipole magnets allow the beam to handle tighter turns.

Other magnets minimize the spread of the particles from the collisions. When it is time to dispose of the particles, they are deflected from the LHC along a straight line towards the beam dump. A "dilution" **magnet** reduces the beam intensity by a factor of 100,000 before the beam collides with a block of concrete and graphite composite for its final stop. **Insertion magnets** are also responsible for beam cleaning, which ensures that stray particles do not come in contact with the LHC's most sensitive components.

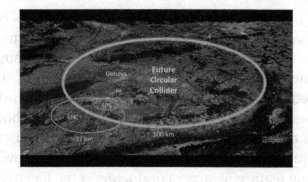

Chapter 5

The Deliberate Suppression of Biomagnetic Healing Throughout History

Subtle Vibrational Energy. Chinese Book of Medicine 3000 b.c. Ka, Chi, Prana, Jesus Heals, The Flexner Report of 1910. Paracelsus. Franz Anton Messmer. Rudolph Steiner, Nikola Tesla. Dr. Randolph Stone, Dr. Goiz & Dr. Luis Garcia

Early records of scientifically advanced civilizations tell us that magnetic forces have long been prized for their restorative properties. Ancient Greece discovered the very first natural magnet in the form of the lodestone, and Hippocrates, the father of medicine, noted its healing powers. The Egyptians, too, described the divine powers of the magnet in their writings, and Cleopatra frequently adorned herself with magnetic jewelry to preserve youthfulness.

Subtle Energy Terms

Chi Ki Vital Life Force Universal Energy

Prana Orgone Akasha Spirit Aether

Source Field Od Nuetrinos Gravity Field

Tesla Waves Scalar Waves Higgs Field

Longitudinal Waves

Cleopatra used a natural magnet (lodestone) to wear on her forehead. It was intended to keep her skin youthful, as a headache reliever, sleeping aid, or maybe to slow down the aging process. Another good reason could have been to stimulate the pineal gland in the brain to release melatonin.

Chinese manuscripts dating back thousands of years describe the Eastern belief that the *life force, termed "qi", is generated by the earth's magnetic field.* Today, many believe that certain places on earth, such as Lourdes, France, and Sedona, Arizona, owe their healing powers to naturally high levels of this qi, or *biomagnetic energy.* The very first book on magnetism was also the first book on medical healing written 3,000 years ago titled, "The Yellow Book of Chinese Medicine".

They're so old the real discovery of magnetism is extremely of a legend. It becomes stated that approximately 4000 years ago, a shepherd named Magnes to become out herding his sheep when his metallic workforce and the nails in his shoes stuck to a black rock. That black rock becomes magnetite and it contained lodestone. Since then, our use of magnets has developed in hundreds of different methods.

The use of laying-on-of-hands to heal human illness dates back thousands of years in human history. Evidence for its use in ancient Egypt is found in the Ebers Papyrus dated at about 1552 b.c. This document describes the use of laying on of hands healing for medical treatment. Four centuries before the birth of Christ, the Greeks used Therapeutic Touch therapy in their Asklepian temples for healing the sick. The writings of Aristophanes detail the use of laying-on-of-hands in Athens to restore a blind man's sight and return fertility to a barren woman.

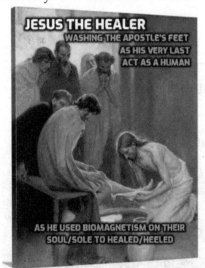

"THE" KJV Bible has many references to the laying-on-of-hands for both medical and spiritual applications. It is known that many of the miraculous healings of Jesus were done by the laying-on-of-hands. Jesus is said to have spoken, " These things that I do, so can you do and more" Laying-on-of-hands healing was considered part of the work of the early Christian ministry as much as preaching and administering these sacraments. In the early Christian church, laying-on-of-hands was combined with the sacramental use of holy water and oil.

Could this be why we use the words "heal" to use some ones heals to heal, just like Jesus did? Or why we say "soul" referencing the *soles of our feet* that ground us to Earth consciousness. Fact is that rubber soles on tennis shoes was introduced to the world with Nike, Converse and Reebok beginning in the early 1960's and disconnected us from Earth Consciousness with the rubber soles..(to disconnect our souls!). This was celebrated with the Tavistock written Beatles song and album named, "Rubber Soul" in released in 1964.

In Europe the healing ministry was carried on as the royal touch. Kings of several European countries were purportedly successful incurring diseases such as tuberculosis (scrofula) by laying-on-of-hands. In England, this method of healing began with Edward the Confessor, lasted for seven centuries, and ended with the reign of the skeptical William IV. Many of the early attempts at laying-on-of-hands healing seemed to be predicated upon a belief either in the powers of Jesus, or the king, or a particular healer. There were other contemporary medical theorists who felt that special vital forces and influences in nature were the mediators of these healing effects. A number of early researchers into the mechanisms of healing theorized on the likely magnetic nature of the energies involved. One of the earliest proponents of a magnetic vital force of nature was the controversial physician Theophrastus Bombastus von Hohenheim, otherwise known as Paracelsus (1493-1541).

Paracelsus, a physician and alchemist, was born in Switzerland in 1493. He was the first to propose that illnesses were caused by external substances (the concept of disease), not imbalances in the body's "humors" (the dominant theory at the time). He recommended using sulfur, mercury, and other substances to treat diseases. Paracelsus had a notion of a "life force" in nature and the human body, which he called archaeus (meaning "ancient"). He treated illnesses by replenishing the archaeus with the energy found in certain herbs and foods. Paracelsus advocated using magnets to energize and influence the body's life force to start the healing process, treating everything from inflammation to diarrhea to epilepsy. In the middle 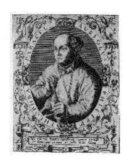 ages, doctors used magnets to treat arthritis, poisoning, gout, baldness, clean wounds and retrieve iron containing objects from the body, like arrowheads. In 1600, William Gilbert, court physician to Elizabeth I of England, published the first scientific treatise on magnetism, "De Magnete".

Paracelsus wandered throughout Europe and the Middle East studying with alchemists. He valued the common sense of common people more than the dry teachings of scientists and stressed nature's healing power. Such broad thinking irritated the authorities, and eventually Paracelsus was forced to flee.

This book summarized the current knowledge about magnetism, showing, for instance, that steel holds a magnetic charge better than iron and that there is a distinction between magnetism and electricity. Gilbert was the first to describe the Earth as a huge magnet with magnetic poles close to the geographic north and south poles. He also confirmed that use of the lodestone could be "beneficial in many diseases of the human system". (The term lodestone for magnetized stones is from the Middle Ages, when the lodestone -- "guiding stone" -- was used in compasses by sailors as a navigational tool.)

Fran Anton Mesmer ~ aka "Mesmerized" (1734-1815)

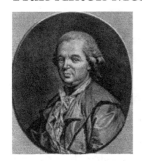
The development in 18th century Europe of carbon-steel permanent magnets, more powerful than lodestones, renewed curiosity in the healing powers of magnets. Maximillian Hell, a professor of astronomy at the University of Vienna, was one of those interested. He claimed several cures using steel magnets. A friend of Hell's, Franz Anton Mesmer, borrowed Hell's magnets to treat a woman suffering from mental illness. He claimed success and began promoting his theory of "animal magnetism." The theory was sufficiently put down after a special commission established by King Louis XVI concluded that all the observed effects of the healing through the use of magnets or items that had been "magnetized" could be attributed to **the power of suggestion**.

Around 1800, Alessandro Volta constructed the first battery (made of silver, moist cardboard, and zinc), which produced a small, steady electric current. Further experiments with electricity by Andre-Marie Ampere, Michael Faraday, and others, established the link between magnetism and electricity. Faraday demonstrated that a ***magnet in motion could produce magnetricity*** and that the flow of electricity produces a magnetic field. This was confirmed by Scottish scientist James Maxwell, who showed that light was an electromagnetic phenomenon as well.

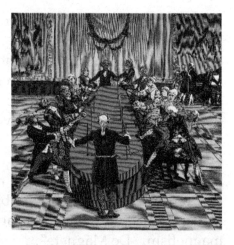

Animal magnetism was all the rage in eighteenth-century Europe, and its star Franz Friedrich Anton Mesmer, a captivating German physician, had celebrity status. His theory claimed that a special kind of imperceptible magnetic fluid pervaded the universe and that most if not all diseases were caused by an abnormal flow of this fluid inside the body. At first, Mesmer's therapeutic technique consisted of waiving magnets around his patients after making them swallow iron filings. He later would forego the swallowing metal stage and also the magnets: he discovered that simply using his hands or other objects was just as effective. After such so-called "passes" the patient would go into a kind of trance state, then faint, convulse, shake, and so on (what would be aptly named a "crisis"). Ideally, after all this evidently flow-inducing activity, they would be healed.

By 1778, having fallen into considerable royal disfavor, Mesmer moved to Paris in a shroud of fame and controversy. Despite the opposition of the medical profession, who denied him a medical license, he partnered up with the respectable and licensed Charles Deslon, personal physician to the brother of King Louis XVI. Mesmer again ended up establishing a stupendously popular clinical practice, winning the favor of many highly influential people. In fact, it only took a few years for animal magnetism to grow into something close to an obsession among the French.

Soon Mesmer and a few disciples started offering magnetic group séances. By the mid-1780s mesmerism had become such a craze that concerned Parisian physicians persuaded the king to establish a royal commission to investigate its claims. The degree to which said craze was lucrative and the rate at which regular medical clinics were losing traffic may, of course, have played a role here. Admittedly, we can sympathize with the patients who deemed that magnetic séances compared favorably with the more mainstream practices of bloodletting and leeching.

Benjamin Franklin was in France as the first US ambassador with a mission to ensure an official alliance against its arch nemesis, the British. On account of his fame as a great man of science in general and his experiments on one such invisible force — electricity — in particular, Franklin was **appointed as head of the French Royal Commission** (*so why was BF named head of a foreign country's commission?*). The investigating team also included the chemist Antoine-Laurent Lavoisier, the astronomer Jean-Sylvain Bailly, and the doctor

Joseph-Ignace Guillotin. It is a curious fact of history that both Lavoisier and Bailly were later executed by the guillotine — the device attributed to their fellow commissioner. The revolution also, of course, brought the same fate to King Louis XVI and his Mesmer-supporting wife Marie Antoinette.

To get magnetism banned by 'science', the commissioners figured that the cures might be affected by one of two possible mechanisms: psychological suggestion (what they refer to as "imagination") or some actual physical magnetic action. Mesmer and his followers claimed it was the magnetic fluid, so that served as the experimental condition if you like. Continuing with the modern analogies, suggestion would then represent a rudimentary placebo control condition. So to test animal magnetism, they came up with two kinds of trials to try and separate the two possibilities: either the research subject is being magnetized but does not know it (magnetism without imagination) or the subject is not being magnetized but thinks that they are (imagination without magnetism). Perhaps unsurprisingly, the commissioners concluded that imagination alone could produce the same striking effects as mesmerism. Furthermore, animal magnetism by itself was completely toothless and impotent. It is admirable that Deslon himself seems to have acknowledged the power of the commissioners' approach and accepted the main findings to do with the existence of this "magnetic fluid". However, even if it proved to be nothing more than imagination, he insisted on its clinical utility. Mesmerism was very much in line with the latest scientific developments. In some ways, exciting experiments with invisible forces — electricity, magnetism, wondrous gases like hydrogen and helium — defined the era. Unlike the occultists of the previous ages, Mesmer was striving to give his practices a rational scientific as opposed to a religious flavor. Indeed, although the magnetic fluid part did not work out, in an important sense, animal magnetism marked the beginnings of hypnosis and psychological suggestion, hence the term "mesmerized" to confuse and conflate the true healing power of magnetism. He was not a quack and Benjamin Franklin and the Royal Academy of Sciences buried him and his findings calling him a "charlatan" and "womanizer" to discredit him.

Here is just some of Mr. Mesmer's findings that prove he was no "Quack":

1. A responsive influence exists between the heavenly bodies, the earth, and animated bodies.

2. A fluid universally diffused, so continuous as not to admit of a vacuum, incomparably subtle, and naturally susceptible of receiving, propagating, and communicating all motor disturbances, is the means of this influence.

3. This reciprocal action is subject to mechanical laws, with which we are not as yet acquainted.

4. Alternative effects result from this action, which may be considered to be a flux and reflux.

5. This reflux is more or less general, more or less special, more or less compound, according to the nature of the causes which determine it.

6. It is by this action, the most universal which occurs in nature, that the exercise of active relations takes place between the heavenly bodies, the earth, and its constituent parts.

7. The properties of matter and of organic substance depend on this action.

8. The animal body experiences the alternative effects of this agent, and is directly affected by its insinuation into the substance of the nerves.

9. Properties are displayed, analogous to those of the magnet, particularly in the human body, in which diverse and opposite poles are likewise to be distinguished, and these may be communicated, changed, destroyed, and reinforced.

10. Even the phenomenon of declination may be observed.

11. This property of the human body which renders it susceptible of the influence of heavenly bodies, and of the reciprocal action of those which environ it, manifests its analogy with the magnet, and this has decided me to adopt the term of animal magnetism.

12. The action and virtue of animal magnetism, thus characterized, may be communicated to other animate or inanimate bodies. Both of these classes of bodies, however, vary in their susceptibility.

13. Experiments show that there is a diffusion of matter, subtle enough to penetrate all bodies without any considerable loss of energy.

14. This action and virtue may be strengthened and diffused by such bodies.

15. Its action takes place at a remote distance, without the aid of any intermediary substance.

16. It is, like light, increased and reflected by mirrors.

17. It is communicated, propagated, and increased by sound.

18. This magnetic virtue may be accumulated, concentrated, and transported.

19. I have said that animated bodies are not all equally susceptible; in a few instances they have such an opposite property that their presence is enough to destroy all the effects of magnetism upon other bodies.

20. This opposite virtue likewise penetrates all bodies: it also may be communicated, propagated, accumulated, concentrated, and transported, reflected by mirrors, and propagated by sound. This does not merely constitute a negative, but a positive opposite virtue.

21. The magnet, whether natural or artificial, is like other bodies susceptible of animal magnetism, and even of the opposite virtue: in neither case does its action on fire

and the needle [of a compass] suffer any change, and this shows that the principle of animal magnetism essentially differs from that of mineral magnetism.

22. This system sheds new light upon the nature of fire and of light, as well as on the theory of attraction, of flux and reflux, of the magnet and of electricity.

23. It teaches us that the magnet and artificial electricity have, with respect to diseases, properties common to a host of other agents presented to us by nature, and that if the use of these has been attended by some useful results, they are due to animal magnetism.

24. These facts show, in accordance with the practical rules I am about to establish, that this principle will cure nervous diseases directly, and other diseases indirectly. By its aid the physician is enlightened as to the use of medicine, and may render its action more perfect, and can provoke and direct salutary crises, so as to completely control them.

25. In communicating my method, I shall, by a new theory of matter, demonstrate the universal utility of the principle I seek to establish.

26. Possessed of this knowledge, the physician may judge with certainty of the origin, nature, and progress of diseases, however complicated they may be; he may hinder their development and accomplish their cure without exposing the patient to dangerous and troublesome consequences, irrespective of age, temperament, and sex. Even women in a state of pregnancy, and during parturition, may reap the same advantage.

27. This doctrine will finally enable the physician to decide upon the health of every individual, and of the presence of the diseases to which he may be exposed. In this way the art of healing may be brought to absolute perfection.

"If you want to find the secrets of the universe, think in terms of energy, frequency and vibration." ~ Nikola Tesla

Tesla Medicine

Few people know Nikola Tesla for his medical inventions that involved the use of magnetism and light to treat a wide variety of disease. Medical textbooks at this time included magnetism and electricity as therapeutic alternatives for mental disorders in particular and other conditions as well. It was recommended for convulsions, insomnia, migraine, fatigue, arthritis, and pain

Nikola Tesla was a master of resonance – the vibrational properties of the solid, liquid and

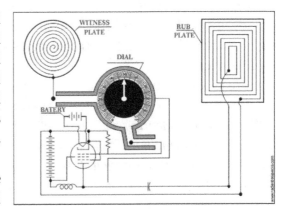

gaseous substance of matter. He understood how physical vibrations of the body could be used as a medicine to treat the human condition. Tesla won the war of currents and a place in history with his AC power distribution system, but his ventures into free wireless energy failed because investors felt it could not be monetized effectively. The ever-popular use of Tesla's magnetism with his radionics devices in western medicine fell to the wayside with the introduction of the AMA, the FDA and patented drugs that could turn a healthy profit for its corporate shareholders.

In a similar fashion, Tesla's electromagnetic medical marvels brought healing fields to the patient via his Tesla coil. The devices would emit oscillating waves of various frequencies consisting of low frequency pulsing magnetic fields to treat pain, acoustic vibration machines to detoxify organs of the body, high frequency cancer killing radio waves and ultra-high frequency ultraviolet light to create ozone to deactivate viruses.

Electricians rushed out to build or purchase these machines and without any medical training started to use them on patients. The Electrotherapeutic Association was formed in Buffalo with chapters in Hamilton and Toronto because electrical power became available to public and private hospitals that were in close proximity to Tesla's generators at Niagara Falls. It is not disclosed how the energy from Niagra Falls was transferred but hospitals in Buffalo became famous worldwide by offering Tesla's magnetic healing treatments and cures for the most serious of diseases and they could boast a very high success rate. However, since the patents for the methods that were used on these devices were practically unenforceable, and Tesla was not interested in defending them either. These devices, known as Radionic machines, were medical devices capable of broadcasting a special healing field to the patient **– even if they were not present in the room.** Medically trained doctors complained to Congress about these devices and formed the American Medical Association to organize the practice of licensed medicine in favor of the newly created Rockefeller Medicine establishment.

The FDA Food and Drug Administration was formed to regulate the use of drugs and energy based medical devices. Manufactures now had to prove their drugs and medical devices worked before they could be sold to the public. This became a rigorous costly procedure that required the help of independent universities to conduct the studies, and since you could not patent frequencies of electricity – few companies decided to license their devices.

Here is an example of a letter that was sent to a popular newspaper by his assistant. Detroit Free Press dated February 16th, 1896:

"While experimenting with a novel contrivance, constituting in its simplest form a vibrating mechanical system, in which from the nature of the construction the applied force is always in resonance with the natural period, I frequently exposed my body to continued mechanical vibrations. As the elastic force can be made as large as desired, and the applied force used be very small, great

weights, half a dozen persons, for instance, may be vibrated with great rapidity by a comparatively small apparatus.

I observed that such intense mechanical vibrations produce remarkable physiological effects. They affect powerfully the condition of the stomach, undoubtedly promoting the process of digestion and relieving the feeling of distress, often experienced in consequence of the imperfect function of the organs concerned in the process. They have a strong influence upon the liver, causing it to discharge freely, similarly to an application of a cathartic. They also seem to affect the glandular system, notably in the limbs; also, the kidneys and bladder, and more or less influence the whole body. When applied for a longer period they produce a feeling of immense fatigue, so that a profound sleep is induced.

The excessive tiring of the body is generally accompanied by nervous relaxation, but there seems to be besides a specific action on the nerves.

These observations, though incomplete, are, in my own limited judgment, nevertheless positive and unmistakable, and in view of this and of the importance of further investigation of the subject by competent men I prepared about a year ago a machine with suitable adjustments for varying the frequency and amplitude of the vibrations, intending to give it to some medical faculty for investigation.

An American who became interested in magnetic healing, Daniel David Palmer, opened Palmer's School of Magnetic Cure in Iowa in the 1890s. His ideas developed into the system of hands-on therapy known today as chiropractic. Others focused on using hand gestures to heal people without actually touching them. This type of therapy was reborn as therapeutic touch.

> *"The day science begins to study non-physical phenomena; it will make more progress in one decade than in all the previous centuries of its existence."*
> – Nikola Tesla 1856-1943

Tesla's medical inventions gradually disappeared from western medicine after the AMA decided to omit them from the course curriculum textbooks that doctors used to pass their exam to legally practice medicine. Eventually, doctors were only trained to prescribe FDA approved prescription drugs and specialists in the human anatomy were taught the best practices in surgery. All electricians and medical doctors that held onto the practice of "therapeutics" such as magnetic field therapy, light therapy, and

Flexner Report : 100 Years

- Published in June, 1910
- Brother of the President of the Rockerfeller Institute
- Reformed medical education
- Modeled after John Hopkins
  - Which was modeled on Germany
- Schools eagerly cooperated in survey hoping for funds

hydrotherapy were considered to be "quacks." Hospitals could not purchase unlicensed machines for therapy and what remained in the way of electrical appliances was mainly used for Xray diagnostics. In general, electricity could be used to diagnose the patient – but magnetic fields were officially deemed to have no effect on the body. Tesla's healing machines were eventually removed from all western medical textbooks.

In the early years of the American empire, when there was still a free market in the medical field, there were many thriving homeopathic hospitals and medical colleges. Over a century ago the Carnegie and Rockefeller foundations decided to engineer the medical curriculum through their grants and donations to the many different medical schools they deemed could be profitable for their associated businesses. As they have done with most facets of American society, they decided that they would reform medical education in America to suit their financial desires. There were many different types of medical schools from homeopathic and herbal, to what we know today as modern western medicine. The Rockefeller and Carnegie foundations sought to patent the petrochemical medical education as the sole practice in the United States. The natural health colleges were not pushing enough chemical drugs, and those drugs were primarily owned by the Carnegies and the Rockefellers.

So out came the authorized preordained Flexner Report, funded by the two foundations, that called on American medical schools to enact higher admission and graduation standards, and in so many words, stated that it was far too easy to open a medical school. This report was used to shift from holistic to pharmaceutical practice. The American Medical Association, who were evaluating the various medical colleges, made it their job to target and shut down the larger more respected homeopathic medical colleges. Carnegie and Rockefeller began to immediately shower hundreds of millions of dollars on the medical schools that focused on teaching drug intensive medicine.

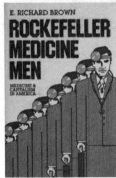

Carnegie and Rockefeller made sure they had their own staff appointed to high positions on the board of directors of these schools. They made sure these schools were teaching the curriculum they dictated, or they would not "donate" the millions that the schools so obviously wanted. Over time they began to fill these boards with members who were literally on the payroll. Once they had entire control of the board, the curriculum of these schools began to swing completely in the sole direction of pharmaceutical drugs which were exclusively sold by Carnegie and Rockefeller, and it has remained that way ever since.

Predictably, the schools that had the funding of these foundations turned out the "recognized" doctors that were taught to push pharmaceutical drugs instead of holistic treatments, even if the holistic treatment could work better, or would cost less. By 1925, 10,000 herbalists were out of business, and *by 1940 over 1500 chiropractors were prosecuted for practicing quackery.* The 22 homeopathic medical schools that flourished in the 1900s dwindled down to just two by 1923, and **by 1950 all the schools teaching homeopathy**

were closed. In the end if a doctor did not graduate from a Flexner approved medical school, he or she could not find a job. Most doctors today do not even realize they are lap dogs of the pharmaceutical industry.

While western medicine was seeing a gradual progression towards a healthcare system based upon patented medicines, Tesla's medicine had remained and were further improved upon by countries that practiced socialized healthcare where the government paid for the health and wellbeing of the public. Countries of the former Soviet Union and the German speaking countries of Europe realized that Tesla's medicine could be used as complimentary therapy. The government of Canada observed the success of cannabis as a natural medicine and along with it came the energy therapies known as "German Medicine" so they eventually lifted the difficult licensing restrictions that were previously placed upon it. In the USA – the FDA has created a new category called "wellness" devices for Tesla's medicine.

Magnet therapy fell into disfavor following World War II with the development of antiobiotics (***anti**=against & **bio** = life or 'against life'*) and biochemistry-based medicine.

The completely made up and fabricated story of how magnets were 'discovered' to heal illness by NASA, (aka NOT A Space Agency), was a fantastical story made up by those that run NASA incorporated at the US Dept. of Defense (Offense). The story goes that the first astronauts returned to earth sick. Their illness was soon attributed to a lack of magnetism in outer space and the problem was subsequently resolved when NASA placed magnets in their space suits and spaceships. This story is impossible since we have never been outside the energy dome above us all at 62 miles above Earth.

So, if true, why has not biomagnetic healing become studied and used in western medicine today and applied? Because, it works and costs little to nothing to use and get results and Western Medi-sin is all about the profits, only about the profits, to "enhance shareholder value" as their main and only business model.

Today, magnet healing protocols are seeing a huge resurgence in application and is an officially approved therapy in over 45 countries worldwide, yet in the United States medical doctors and healers have to be very cautious as not to attract the Medical Mafia Police to shut down this most amazing healing protocol anyone can learn. The overlying threat to Big Pharma drug sales as well as close hospitals and put nearly anyone and everyone out of business in the for profit, never a cure, (can't use the word 'cure'), worst of the worst medical communities worldwide.

The mind-body split occurred in Western tradition during the Renaissance. Scientists asked for the permission of the authorities to examine the body – which was granted on condition that the authorities (the medieval Church) kept the soul. The majority of Western medical scientific tradition then developed with a worldview that excluded the soul. The Newtonian physics of cause and effect became pre-eminent. Tremendous technological advances in the material world were based on newly discovered laws of physics and chemistry.

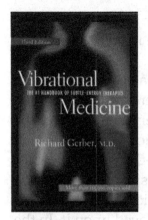

Cultural advances depended on these technological improvements in the visible physical world – and dazzled our eyes to the point that we could forget the existence of the soul, along with the rest of invisible reality. Effectively, much of Western Medicine has looked exhaustively at the hardware of the body, whilst ignoring the software of the circuits of the consciousness (our invisible thoughts and feelings) running on the hardware! Moreover, it may mistake the effects of thoughts and feelings (neurotransmitters and neural impulses) for the causative factors. Pert has published extensively on this. However, even in Western tradition, some of our greatest thinkers have considered the position; it was Leonardo da Vinci who stated in 1499 that: "By the law of the Almighty The body is the work of the soul Which fashions its outward appearance By hammering it from within Like a goldsmith embosses his material. Perhaps, as physics tells us, the whole universe is composed of vibrations dancing in and out of tune with each other, and as Eastern traditions tell us, consciousness underpins and pervades all matter – perhaps we are all aspects of consciousness experiencing life in a human frame. Perhaps we do not live life, but rather life lives through us? ~ Vibrational Medicine by Richard Gerber

Biomag Revisited

"Life is a song. It has its own rhythm of harmony. It is a symphony of all things, which exist in major and minor keys of Polarity. It blends the discords, by opposites, into a harmony that unites the whole into a grand symphony of life. To learn through experience in this life, to appreciate the symphony and lessons of life and to blend with the whole, is the object of being here.

The whole constitution of man must be taken into consideration, not merely the treating of the body as a chemical or mechanical machine." ~ Dr. Randolph Stone

Dr. Randolph Stone (February 26, 1890 – December 9, 1981) was the founder of polarity therapy, a complementary technique of holistic, spiritually based energy healing. He held doctorates in osteopathy, chiropractic, and naturopathy. He had an interest in philosophy and religions, and encountered Ayurvedic philosophy on a trip to India. His background in chiropractic was shaped by his studies of various 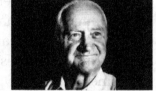 Eastern concepts of energy medicine, including Ayurveda, traditional Chinese medicine, yoga, and reflexology. It was Dr. Stone who coined the definition of 'Polarity Therapy'.

"Polarity therapy is a holistic, energy-based system that includes bodywork, diet, exercise, and lifestyle counseling for the purpose of restoring and maintaining proper energy flows throughout the body.

The underlying concept of polarity therapy is that all energy within the human body is based in electromagnetic force and that disease results from improperly dissipated energy. After determining

the exact source of a patient's energy imbalance, the therapist begins the first of a series of bodywork sessions designed to re channel and release the patient's misdirected prana. This therapy, akin to massage, is based in energetic pressure and involves circulating motions. In performing the regimen, the therapist pays strict attention to the pressure exerted at each location – even to which finger is used to apply pressure at any given point of the patient's anatomy.

This technique, which comprises the central regimen or focal point of polarity therapy is very gentle and is unique to polarity therapy. It typically involves subtle rocking movements and cranial holds to stimulate body energy. Although firm, deep pushing touches are employed in conjunction with the massage technique, the polarity therapist never exerts a particularly forceful contact. To support the bodywork, the therapist often prescribes a diet for the patient, to encourage cleansing and eliminate waste. The precepts of polarity therapy take into consideration specific interactions between different foods and the human energy fields. May this work reach the seekers who are looking for a deeper perspective of a common denominator in the healing art, to push it along in keeping with all the atomic discoveries of today. The health and well-being of the people should not be neglected. It should really be the first concern of the scientists, doctors and educators. Without health and happiness, all our modern conveniences are of little comfort to us."

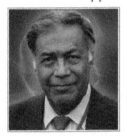

Dr. Isaac Goiz Duran (1941-2021) Father of Modern Day Biomagnetism
Much credit is well deserved to Dr. Goiz and his family from Mexico for bringing modern day biomagnetism to the modern world. In the 1970's, Dr. Randolph Stone laid out in his book, "Polarity Therapy" the means and methods to heal with magnetic energy in great detail and I have never read or seen anywhere where Dr. Goiz has acknowledged the fine work before him of Dr. Stone.

Dr. Goiz did greatly progress modern techniques and knowledge and many, included myself, have benefitted greatly from his deep work in biomagnetic healing. Dr. Goiz successfully treated more than 350.000 patients with Biomagnetism and has trained more than 10,000 medical doctors and other health practitioners from many different countries, mainly South America, America and Europe.

- Physiotherapist – Physical Medicine School at "Americano Británico" Hospital in Mexico, 1964
- Medical Surgeon – "Autónoma de Puebla" University in Mexico, 1984
- General Director and Founder of "Medical Biomagnetism Researching Centre", S.C., 1994
- Bioenergetics Medicine Ph.D, by Oxford International University, England, 1999
- Member of New York Academy of Sciences in USA, 2000

Sadly, Dr. Goiz, when hosting Biomag Healing seminars, mainly only gave presentations in Spanish and required students who traveled great distances to learn Biomag Healing must sign a contract agreeing that they will "never can become teachers of biomagnetism" before they entered the room for the workshop after paying up front and traveling to the teaching site! Why would he do that? Many had no idea they would be required to sign such a solely self-serving document for the Goiz family. The Goiz protocols left it up to each individual to translate and formulate their own healing protocols from Spanish with little help with diagrams or placement help. In addition, Dr. Goiz claims here that he was the first to help and heal a souls at distance, when it is clear from the history of biomag healing that he was not the first. From Jesus to Parcelsus, to Anton Mesmer, before him and even Dr. Randolph Stone, to set the record straight here, he was not the first and has given zero credit to others before him and his family has even attacked others who learned BiomagHealing techniques for their own findings and progression.

From Dr. Goiz's website;

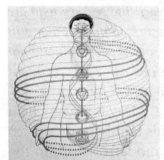

Throughout history it's been proven effective, but he was the first modern biomag healer "The phenomenon that we call Biomagnetic Pair is important for the health of the patient, but in 1993, in April, I spontaneously discovered that the phenomenon that the magnets produce in the presence of distorted charges in the human body can also be produced by the power of thoughts. This is now a phenomenon that is strictly between the mind of the therapist and the biological behavior of the damaged tissue.

And this opens up new possibilities to understanding the pathology, because we are now going into such depth of understanding that we couldn't achieve with simple magnets, obviously. And this opens doors to psychological, emotional, and spiritual problems, and obviously this shatters the constructs of conventional medicine, when we delve into such depths of the human body. So I worked on this for another two years, and in 1995, thanks to the spontaneous cure of a man named Chiro Ayello, he in turn asked me to cure his brother in a town called Piano Sorrento, Italy. This man suffered from such a terrible migraine that he had contemplated suicide. We gave it a try and managed to impact the phenomenon from Mexico to Italy, and for the first time, a patient was cured at a distance. In 1994 the medical Biomagnetism gave a "quantum leap" since Dr. Goiz was able to mentally detect the phenomena of bioenergetic polarization. That is to say, he was able to obtain the shortening of the patient's hemibody without having to do the scan with the negative magnet. It was enough to ask "mentally" about the different points to obtain a physical response. In 1995 Dr. Isaac Goiz Durán was able to perform a complete remote treatment through the phenomenon of bioenergetic induction between Mexico City and the Piano of Sorrento, Italy. Nowadays, remote healing is a function of the bioenergetic pair with these criteria, the depolarization of the altered organs, was achieved since 1988, facing the bioenergetic charges by means of natural magnets superior to 1,000 Gauss. http://bmguide.guiabiomagnetismo.com/pares.htm

Rules of practice from *"Biomagnetic Pair"* by Dr. Isaac Goiz Duran (almost the exact same conclusions that Franz Anton Messmer cited)

1. Biomagnetism is a therapeutic and diagnosis procedure.
2. The positive biomagnetic pole is formed by the presence of hydrogen ions, H+ and/or pathogenic viruses.
3. The negative biomagnetic pole is formed by the presence of free radicals and/or pathogenic bacteria.
4. The biomagnetic poles are in *vibrational and energetic resonance.*
5. The biomagnetic poles are depolarized by the magnetic induction of fields greater than 1,000 gauss.
6. The biomagnetic depolarizationis due to the law of all or nothing.
7. The biomagnetic *depolarization obeys the universal law of charges.*
8. The biomagnetic induction is instantaneous but the charge is exhausted in seconds.
9. The ideal magnetic fields for the induction are between 5,000 and 10,000 gauss.
10. When the biomagnetic poles are impacted? *the pathogenic viruses lose their genetic information and the bacteria lose their favourable alkaline medium which is important for their metabolism and reproduction.*
11. The positive biomagnetic poles are asymptomatic, they cannot be detected by other conventional system of diagnosis nor they can be healed or corrected by any other therapeutic or drug method.
12. The negative biomagnetic poles are symptomatic and they can be healed and corrected by other medical procedures or drug method.
13. In a Normal Energetic Level (NEL) any pathogenic microorganisms cannot be generated, but they can be manifested by themselves and by their metabolites.
14. Natural magnets of medium intensity are not toxic nor they can produce iatrogenic effects, especially when they are applied in a dual manner.
15. Natural magnets of medium intensity do not alter the cellular or tissue entropy. They only put it in order.
16. The hydrogen bridge cannot be broken by magnetism but it can be broken by electricity, heat and extreme atomic radiation.
17. The regular BMP's identify *pathogenic microorganisms whether they are viruses, bacteria, fungi or parasites.*
18. The special BMP's identify tissue alterations not supported by pathogenic microorganisms.
19. The dysfunctional BMP's identify internal gland alterations and their hormonal production.

20. The reservoir BMP's identify organs or tissues which support viruses, bacteria, fungi and parasites which are potentially pathogenic, for an indefinite time.

21. In the north hemisphere of the earth, the negative poles of the BMP's tend to be established in the right half of the body. The opposite happens in the southern hemisphere.

22. Common diseases are produced by a single BMP. *Complex diseases are the result of an association of various BMP's.*

"Science and art belong to the whole world, and the barriers of nationality vanish before them" – Johann Wolfgang von Goethe (1749-1832)

Dr. Luis Garcia

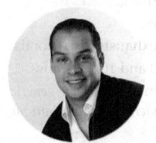

• Bachelor of Science Degree in Biology from Boston College in 1997 where his genetic research landed him in an international scientific publication (Development, 1997) as an undergraduate.

• Medical Degree Universidad de la Sabana in Bogota, Colombia in 2005 and served as Medical Director

• Chief Science Officer of "Salud Futura" Clinic in Bogotá, Colombia Also has studied and worked in the fields of Neurofeedback, Neural therapy, Ozone therapy, Homotoxicology, Neurolinguistic Programming, Chelation therapy, DMSO therapy, Bioenergetics, Nutritional therapies, traditional western medicine and Biomagnetism.

Dr. Garcia honed his Complementary and Alternative Medicine (CAM) skills by learning from top experts in the field. He has spent many years traveling throughout the US, Mexico, Cuba, Ecuador and Colombia mastering an extensive variety of CAM techniques. His stated goal is to stabilize the body's pH and stimulate the immune system through the use of magnets and bioenergetic therapies, which assist the body to regain its self-healing electromagnetic balance naturally. Dr Garcia is recognized in Colombia as one of the leading CAM medical experts in areas including cardiovascular disease, gastrointestinal disorders, diabetes, chronic fatigue, autoimmune disease, cancer and other concerns associated with aging.

"I admire, respect, and thank Dr. Isaac Goiz Duran for his "Nobel prize worthy" genius work and effort. Dr. Goiz's method is unique and so are his discovered pairs and his therapy continues to evolve. This is only the beginning of a transformational healing wave that is moving across the earth. I want to be part of that healing medical movement!", Dr. Garcia declares.

Dr. Garcia has trained in Biomagnetism and Bioenergy work with Dr. Izaac Goiz Duran, Dr. David Goiz Martinez, Dr. Miguel Ojeda Rios, Antonio Salas PhD, Jorge Tapia (Mexico), Gustavo Guayasamin (Ecuador), Carlos Zamora (Chile)(Resecado), Veturián Arana

(SAAMA), Dr. Armando Solarte and John Grinder (NLP, Neurolinguistic Programming). Dr. Garcia has been able to combine his Medical knowledge and extensive research experience with his Biomagnetism and Bioenergy work to discover new Biomagnetism pairs associated with Lyme disease and its co-infections.

He began learning about biomagnetic healing by taking over 20 courses given by Dr. Goiz and then brought the knowledge to his healing business in New York and New Jersey. Though Dr. Garcia is booked out as long as 8 months with souls needing his expert biomag healing protocols, he indevoured to bring the greatest healing protocol to the everyone so that eventually we can "Heal the World".

Through the past 14 years of exclusive focus on biomag healing, assisting to heal thousands of souls, his healing protocol is light years beyond anyone else's these days and he willingly shares with all who take his workshop. His testimonials and track record of healing is well chronicled and he willingly gives his time to help us newbies to biomag healing become more effective and more proficient where he gives up his weekends with his family to help us with his "Hands on Healing" seminars. Hopefully, by this reading, he will have published his online Beyond Biomag Healing Intensive Workshop" so more can learn from the Master himself as well as get updates as to the latest healing protocols dealing with so many internal and external toxic issues we face today.

The Return to Spiritual Science of Healing

Rudolph Steiner (1861-1925) was an intuit and clairvoyant, who founded the Waldorf Schools and wrote the book, "The Spiritual Science of Medicine" He spoke in his lecture titled, "**Young Doctors Course: Lecture VII**" about Biomagnetic Healing on the energetic planes of humans that will come to the forefront of Spiritual Science healing in the century to follow, which is NOW!

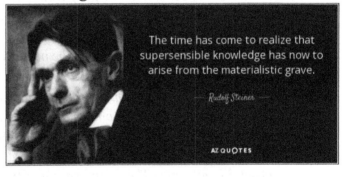

The time has come to realize that supersensible knowledge has now to arise from the materialistic grave.

— *Rudolf Steiner* —

AZ QUOTES

" *The following is also possible. Out of our own astral body, without the patient exerting his own will, we can influence our own etheric body in such a way that our own etheric body works upon the etheric body of the patient in the same way as, in the previous case, the astral body worked. It is in this that healing magnetism consists. The magnetic healer does this unconsciously; he influences his own etheric body with his astral body. Instinctively, he can then so direct the forces he unfolds that as he passes them on to the patient they strengthen the patient's forces. You must realize that if it is to be a question of healing, the magnetic healer must use means that are able, somehow, to bring it about. If we have a patient who is weak, of whose will we can expect nothing, the forces of healing magnetism may sometimes be applied. But I want to say, with emphasis, that magnetic healing forces are pretty problematical and are not equally useful in all cases. The instinctive faculty of activating one's own astral body in order thereby to influence one's own etheric body and then work over into the etheric body of the patient — this instinctive faculty is an individual one. There are people in whom it is strong, others in whom it is weak, others who do not possess it at all. There are people who are, by nature, magnetic healers — certainly there are. But the important thing is this, that the faculty is, as a rule, of limited duration. The natural magnetic healers have this magnetism, as it is called. When they begin to apply it, it may work very well; after a time it begins to wane, and later on it often happens that magnetic healers, after this faculty has died down in them, go on acting as if they still had it, and then charlatanism begins.*

*This is the precarious element when magnetic healing becomes a profession. This kind of healing really cannot be made into a profession. That is what must be said about it. The process of magnetic healing — when a person has the faculty for it — is only unconditionally effective when it **is carried out with genuine compassion for the patient**, a compassion that goes right down into one's organism. If you practice magnetic healing with a real love for the patient, then it cannot be done as a profession. If real love exists it will always be able to lead to something good, if no trouble arises from another side. But it can only be done on occasions, when karma leads us to a person whom we are able, out of love, to help; then the outer sign may be a laying on of the hand, or a stroking and then what is happening is that the astral body is passing on its forces to the etheric body which then works upon the ether body of the other person.*

Out of our own astral body, without the patient exerting his own will, we can influence our own etheric body in such a way that our own etheric body works upon the etheric body of the patient in the same way as, in the previous case, the astral body worked. It is in this that healing magnetism consists. The magnetic healer does this unconsciously; he influences his own etheric body with his astral body. Instinctively, he can then so direct the forces he unfolds that as he passes them on to the patient they strengthen the patient's forces. You must realize that if it is to be a question of healing, the magnetic healer must use means that are able, somehow, to bring it about. If we have a patient who is weak, of whose will we can expect nothing, the forces of healing magnetism may sometimes be applied.

But I want to say, with emphasis, that magnetic healing forces are pretty problematical and are not equally useful in all cases. The instinctive faculty of activating one's own astral body in order thereby to influence one's own etheric body and then work over into the etheric body of the patient — this instinctive faculty is an individual one. There are people in whom it is strong, others in whom it is weak, others who do not possess it at all. There are people who are, by nature, magnetic healers — certainly there are. But the important thing is this, that the faculty is, as a rule, of limited duration. The natural magnetic healers have this magnetism, as it is called. When they begin to apply it, it may work very well; after a time it begins to wane, and later on it often happens that magnetic healers, after this faculty has died down in them, go on acting as if they still had it, and then charlatanism begins. "

"https://wn.rsarchive.org/Medicine/YoungDoctors/19240108p01.html

Chapter 6

BiomagAGriculture ~ Super Grow
*More*Stronger*Faster

B enefits of the application of irrigation with Magnetic treatments in agriculture. Magnetite. Structured Water. Magnetized Garden Beds

Rediscovering nature's secret force of growth:

How to farm properly as god intended" ~ ***Phillip Callahan*** ~

Benefits of the Application of Irrigation With Magnetic Treatments In Agriculture:

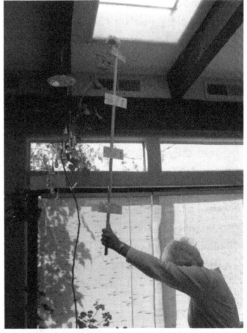

1. IMPROVES the capacity of root absorption.
2. SOLUBILIZES the dissolvable fraction of the soil and clays.
3. OPTIMIZES the yield of fertilizers in the crops.
4. INCREASES the capacity of the field, making it more usable by the roots.
5. REDUCES the formation of lumps (balance between the solution of soil and clays, thus increasing the solubility of soil water)
6. ELIMINATES the deposits of salts, making it easier for plants to extract nutrients more effectively.
7. ACCELERATES the maturation cycle of plants and crops, due to the water dynamics between the clay-humic complex and soil solution.
8. AVOID and ELIMINATES calcareous incrustations and the deposit of algae in drip and sprinkler irrigation
9. DECREASES the irrigation time, because the roots more quickly absorb the nutrients.
10. AVOIDS burned tips, by having the calcium salts not adhere to the leaves.

- There are several hypotheses that try to explain the phenomenon but there are also unknown aspects:
- Hypothesis based on modifications in the water itself
- Hypotheses based on the interaction of the electromagnetic fields with the ions present in aqueous solutions
- Hypothesis based on the interaction of electromagnetic fields on the colloidal ferromagnetic particles.

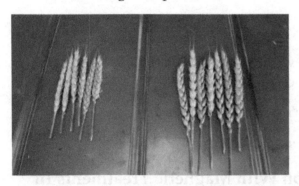

In particular, the magnetic treatment of recycled water and 3000 ppm saline water respectively increased celery yield by 12% and 23% and water productivity by 12% and 24%. For snow peas, there were 7.8%, 5.9% and 6.0% increases in pod yield with magnetically treated potable water, recycled water and 1000 ppm saline water, respectively. The water productivity of snow peas increased by 12%, 7.5% and 13% respectively for magnetically treated potable water, recycled water and 1000 ppm saline water. On the other hand, there was no beneficial effect of magnetically treated irrigation water on the yield and water productivity of peas. There was also non-significant effect of magnetic treatment of water on the total water used by any of the three types of vegetable plants tested in this study.

Magnetic Treatment of Irrigation Water: Evaluation of its Effects on Vegetable Crop Yield and Water

Paramagnetism. Dr Callahan's more recent research and discoveries in relation to paramagnetism are only just beginning to achieve widespread acceptance. Paramagnetism in agriculture is a powerful growth force which enhances root development and stimulates the multiplication of micro-organisms. Dr. Callahan describes paramagnetism as a physical force which is beneficial to plant growth. It is "the alignment of a force field in one direction by a substance in a magnetic field". He tells us that with his research that farmers should consider using paramagnetic rock material on their soils.

Mr. Callahan states that the north magnetic monopoles come in and are attracted to the plants, tree leaves and green vegetation while the south magnetic monopoles are attracted to the soil, rocks and stones. In normal plant growth the south magnetic monopoles migrate through the soil to the roots of the plants. At the same time the north magnetic monopoles are attracted to the plant leaves. This combination gives the plants a magnetic dipole charge.

As a result the south magnetic monopoles in the soil are attracted to the roots of the plants and, as Callahan says, the roots act as wave guides for the south poles to run up through plant stem to recombine with their former mates, the north poles, that are waiting for them in the plant leaves. This recombination releases a large amount of energy that the plant uses to support the photosynthesis process.

Mr. Callahan has proven time and again that plants grow better and stronger and need less water when planted in paramagnetic soil. Adding even a small amount of magnetite and or magnetic water to the soil has a very similar effect but even more so, on plant growth as that of paramagnetic soil alone.

Furthering the optimialized growing environment should/could include biodynamic farming techniques developed by Rudolph Steiner, which we will cover later in this chapter.

Magnetic monopoles are attracted to the soil and, in turn, run through the plant roots, up the stems and through the branch to the leaves to find their mates, the north magnetic monopoles. Viola! More accelerated plant growth which is directly due to the reunion of both north and south magnetic monopoles and the energy that is released with their reunion. Elegant, simple, natural and beautifully reconnecting to earth, air, soil and water through energetic reunion, balance and harmony, which plants respond in kind to grow super produce, lengthen growing cycle and magnetize the soil.

BiomagAG Applications

1) **Sowing Seeds**. Put a red magnet on the seed packages, red against seeds before sowing into trays or pots. Red magnet placed face down on seed package for *15-20* minutes. This stimulates root growth, especially the tap root.

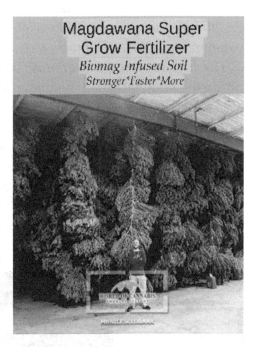

Magdawana Super Grow Fertilizer
Biomag Infused Soil
*Stronger*Faster*More*

2) **Magnetized Structured Water**. Magnetize your water with structured water nozzle, or your main water magnetized will work as well. You can find products to magnetize your water supply at *biomag. com* under products. Creating structured water ionizes the magnetic field properties to purify and enhance optimal water quality that plants thrive on.

3) **Magnetite**. Super Soil enhancer. Miz 4/1 Topsoil to magnetite in both your seed trays and mix with your top soil amendments to your garden beds. You may still be able to buy magnetite on Ebay. Look for the seller from Paradise, CA on ebay or find your own source.

4) **Magnetized Garden Beds**. Ideally, you want to align your garden beds North and South. The idea is to align the magnetic polarities with Earth's magnetic North pole.

Use a compass to determine correct direction. Then, at the bottom of your garden. You then will bury, at the bottom of the garden beds a set of 5 magnets taped together or sealed with beeswax. Then run a galvanized wire around the magnets set into the south end of the bed and run the wire north to the other end. There is a video on how to do this.

https://www.youtube.com/watch?v=S9Go7-Zd1y0

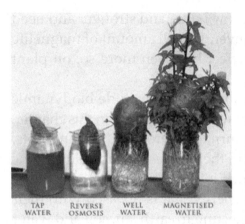

TAP WATER   REVERSE OSMOSIS   WELL WATER   MAGNETISED WATER

Throughout history, farmers have been known to distribute ground-up paramagnetic rock in their fields to revitalize the soil and stimulate plant or crop growth. Paramagnetic rock aka Magnetite, generally directs and amplifies organic energy in a single direction. The organic energy actually converges like a beam as it passes through a medium, such as the ground or air. Hence, this paramagnetic force functions as a magnetic modulator and stimulant for plant growth and increased agricultural output. As will be demonstrated below, the present invention is a paramagnetic-diamagnetic system that can be used to grow plants, as well as provide an organic, biodegradable solution for pest control without polluting the environment or increasing medical risks, and the like.

"My interest in paramagnetism began with a study of sacred places. I visited these sites all over the world – Catholic, Buddhist, Moslem, even Australian Aboriginal sites. I noticed that the plant growth was always better at these places, which always seemed to involve rocks. Further investigation revealed that these rocks were highly paramagnetic". Dr. Callahan

The first reported therapeutic use of magnets involved the grinding up of a naturally occurring material called magnetite and the application of this in poultice form to uncomfortable areas of the body. Magnetite makes for a relatively weak magnet by today's standards. But since the earth's naturally occurring magnetic field was far higher in the past (2 to 3 gauss as opposed to 1/2 gauss today), magnetite crystals may have been stronger at one point in time. Healthy plants emit a different signal than unhealthy plants, and insects are more attracted to the nutritionally deficient plants. The point is that this force was already there. It is there to be harvested. The archaeologists would call this "gathering". Good farming is not synthetic; it must involve working with nature rather than with synthetic poisons. Paramagnetic materials are there to be harvested. Good farming is "gathering".

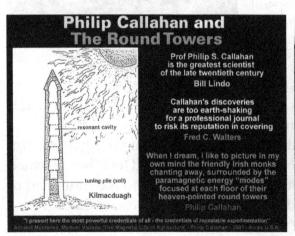

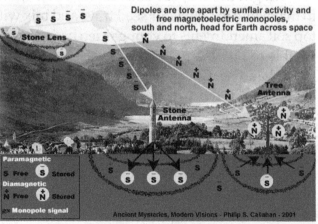

Paramagnetic force is light from rocks for the roots. The rock is actually a transceiver, collecting magnetism from the cosmos and throwing it back out to the roots. If you take a paramagnetic rock and put it into Dr [Fritz-Albert] Popp's lab in Germany and measure it with his instruments which count photons one at a time, you'll find that a highly paramagnetic rock puts out 2,000 to 4,000 photons. If you put that rock with some compost, if you treat it organically, it goes from 2,000 to 4,000 photons to 400,000 photons. Now you are generating a light for roots. Roots are wave-guides, just like the antennae on insects. If you clean off the roots and shine a light on them, they'll wave-guide just like a fibre optic. Soil life is the thing. Paramagnetism works with compost. There may be hundreds of organic growers out there doubling their yields, but when you apply the same material to a dead, chemically farmed soil it won't work. If you don't have a minimum level of organic matter, paramagnetism doesn't work. I've even trialed it at home. Both of my turnip plots have had paramagnetic material added, but one has also had compost. There is no comparison between the growth: compost is the key. You will still need nutrition to benefit from paramagnetism. It's part of a bigger picture. Science is supposed to study nature. When you see something happen, you experiment with it. Then you try to engineer it. This is when the maths comes in, but it should come in after the experiments, not before. Calcium is the most important nutrient, and you won't get a good response from paramagnetic rock dusts if you have ignored your calcium. Nutrients in general won't be available if you don't have enough calcium. Paramagnetism is not a substitute for nutrition. It is something extra.

Structured Water. Structured water is pure water found in nature. It's water from clean springs and streams and the water in fruits and vegetables like cucumbers and melons. Structured water is the optimal source of hydration, energy and vitality because it's the water your cells need to function, heal and repair. Your body was designed to use water as the ultimate fuel.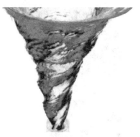

Benefits of Magnetized Water Ingestion
- Better taste
- Reduces acidity and helps regulate the body's pH
- It produces therapeutic effects in the body, especially in the digestive, nervous, and urinary systems
- Helps to clean blocked arteries, normalizes the system, helps create chelating action
- Is beneficial for kidney problems, obesity, gout, and premature aging
- Stimulates brain activity
- Facilitates relaxation and well-being
- Provides more health and vitality

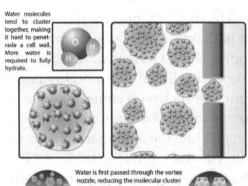

Water molecules tend to cluster together, making it hard to penetrade a cell wall. More water is required to fully hydrate.

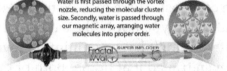

Water is first passed through the vortex nozzle, reducing the molecular cluster size. Secondly, water is passed through our magnetic array, arranging water molecules into proper order.

The Result: Water molecules are properly sorted, easily penetrating the cell wall, requiring less water to produce the desired result, full hydration.

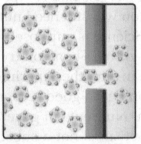

Photographs of tap water frozen crystals and photographs of frozen crystals of the same water after its treatment by the Atlantik and the Medic uran devices

before treatment   after treatment

Photographed by: www.wasserkristall.ch

Plants and the human body share a highly important aspect: each thrives with quality water that has a high level of purity and provides the minerals that create healthy cell rebuilding and growth. Without a high level of purity and/or without bioavailable minerals, we see negative effects. Notice how the city tap water and reverse osmosis water produced severely dehydrated potatoes. The magnetic fields broke down the minerals into smaller clusters, making them easier to absorb. The same effect happens in the human or animal body. During this process of passing water through a high magnetic flux density field the molecules in the water, begin to sort themselves, or self-organize, in the field of the magnets. It's this structuring of the molecules which makes the water more bioavailable to the plants. This is called redox potential, it's a measurement of how much water a plant can soak up. Centripetal spin in the vortex combines with centripetal flux from super-magnets – to produce water molecules stable as more micro cluster, meaning smaller and more spun. This creates absorption, and solubility. Watch as the Super water soaks into the soil visibly faster in your potted plants.

"The analysis of the data collected during the study suggests that the effects of magnetic treatment varied with plant type and the type of irrigation water used, and there were statistically significant increases in plant yield and water productivity (kg of fresh or dry produce per kL of water used). In particular, the magnetic treatment of recycled water and 3000 ppm saline water respectively increased celery yield by 12% and 23% and water productivity by 12% and 24%. For snow peas, there were 7.8%, 5.9% and 6.0% increases in pod yield with magnetically treated potable water, recycled water and 1000 ppm saline water, respectively. The water productivity of snow peas increased by 12%, 7.5%

and 13% respectively for magnetically treated potable water, recycled water and 1000 ppm saline water." ~Basant L. Maheshwari *, School of Natural Science, CRC for Irrigation Futures, Building H3 – Hawkesbury Campus, University of Western Sydney. US Federal Reseach shows- strong magnetic field treatment of water- eliminated need for water softener and decrease pipe build up/scaling.

Implosion Creates, Explosion Destroys

Viktor Shauberger grew up in Austria in the late 1800s in an old growth forest where he studied the movement patterns of water and by the early 1900s he had learned to work with the powers of nature to create inventions like powerful free energy machines, transportation technologies, even levitational devices. Nature never slows down or suffers from entropy; she is always prolifically creating life and sustaining life and recycling life. And nature does this through the movements of water through plants and bodies and ecosystems, right? Water is an integral part in creating and sustaining all life. By understanding the movements of water, Viktor Shauberger was able to uncover the energy-generating principle that sustains everything. And by harnessing that force, he was able to create technologies that work in harmony with the earth instead of against it. He showed that there are two forms of motion in nature — explosive and implosive, or outward and inward. The outward motion is expansive and destructive. It generates heat, pressure, and even death. Its what nature uses when she wants to break down, decompose, decay. It's an important part of nature, but it expends more energy than it creates and can be harmful. Go figure, all of human technology is explosive - its fire based. Combustion engines and nuclear power and coal. Anything that radiates outward, right.

On the other hand, the inward, implosive quality of water produces coolness, suction, powerful vortices, and vitality; it is used to build up and energize and is life-enhancing and life-promoting. Think of the way sap spirals up a tree, the way blood spirals through your veins, the way plants grow in spiral patterns, the way a river courses through its banks in a horizontal spiral. All these vortexes are implosive, energy-generating flows that

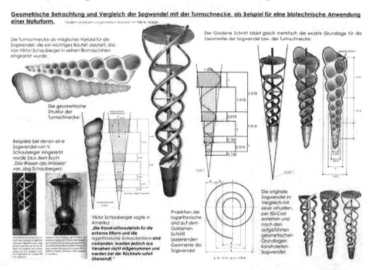

sustain life. If we were to switch our paradigm to implosive, rather than explosive, we could put an end to the drought and destruction on this planet.

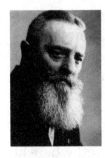

"Protecting the secret of water is a means to protect the interest-power of money. Only in an economy of scarcity can interest thrive. The price of food and the cost of mechanical power would sink to such low levels that speculators would be able to gain nothing from them. Free access to nutrition and mechanical energy are such radical ideas that our concept of the world and all ideologies would be turned upside-down…The secret of water is the capital of Capital — which is why any attempt to reveal it is ruthlessly terminated." ~ *Viktor Schauberger*

So eventually his genius caught the attention of all the wrong people. Hitler met with him in 1934 to discuss the potential of weaponizing water, but he refused to collaborate with Nazis. And his resistance landed him an internment in one of the most horrific of all death camps in the Third Reich — Mauthausen, in Austria. Against his will, he was

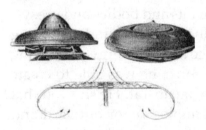

forced to work on a prototype of a gravity-defying flying machine, the Vril-7. That's where he harnessed waters levitational properties to create an anti-gravity device, called a Repulsine. Afterward, the British, Americans, and Russians were all fighting over the spoils of war, especially human resources. And along with scores of other scientists, Schauberger became a natural target. What remained of his work fell into the hands of American and Russian agents. But it was the Americans who took possession of Schauberger himself and held him prisoner and made him disclose his work.

He was taken to NASA through Operation Paperclip where over 4,000 Nazi generals and scientists were brought into the US to run many corporations like the drug company Bayer and top jobs at NASA, including V-2 Buzz bomb "Vunderkind" Werhner Von Bruan to run the Saturn Rocket Program for the faked Apollo missions to the moon. Having no more use for him, they sent him back to Austria when he refused to cooperate and was 'suicided' 5 days later. He told his friends and family that they had stolen his soul. Mr. Schauberger died a broken and penniless man.

Pyramids Are Super Seed Growing Centers

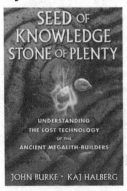

The main premise of this must have book is that many megalithic structures were built to amplify electromagnetic effects in order to increase the fertility and viability of the societies' seed stock. It seems that one of the authors worked in a lab, helping to develop a new technique for enhancing seed growth with controlled showers of electrons. They present scientifically documented evidence that the old-world engineers who built the massive henges, pyramids, mounds and dolmen of the ancient world may well have understood a true secret — lost to modern man until now. These structures were overwhelmingly sited at locations where the local geology magnified naturally occurring electromagnetic fluctuations in the earth's crust and, further, that pyramidal and corbel- roofed stone structures erected at these locations enhanced this effect. They travel to many megalithic sites in different parts of the world, trusty magnetometers and electrostatic voltmeters in hand. From Guatemala to England, Peru to New York State, North Dakota to France, they measure, compile records and make their case.

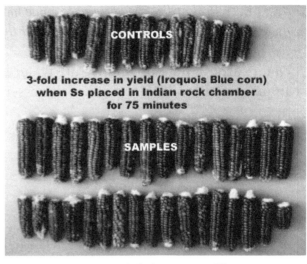

3-fold increase in yield (Iroquois Blue corn) when Ss placed in Indian rock chamber for 75 minutes

In Chapter 3 they discuss the consciousness-altering effects of magnetically anomalous geology, including how it relates to shamanism and dowsing. They seem to be making these points in order to prove that people without instruments could have detected and used those forces to enhance the viability of seeds. Additionally, they reveal that indigenous seeds, when placed at these locations (for various periods of time, depending upon the type of seed) show significant increases in growth rate and yield when subsequently planted — as well as increased resistance to plant stressors (lack of sunlight and/or drought conditions). Such results would have been of enormous importance to ancient peoples and the authors suggest that the monument-builders not only knew these facts, but deliberately chose these sites and structure-shapes in order to insure their culture's food production.

Most cells contain between 70 and 80 percent water. According to Margulis and Sagan (1986): *'The concentrations of salts in both sea-water and blood are, for all practical purposes, identical. The proportions of sodium, potassium, and chloride in our tissues are intriguingly similar to those of the world-wide ocean.... we sweat and cry what is basically seawater"*. Without water, a cell cannot function; as De Duve (1984)

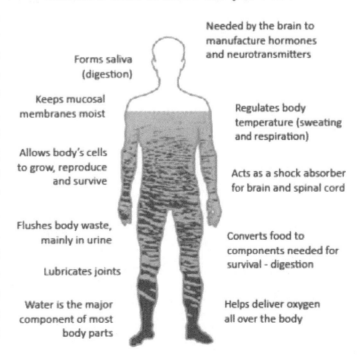

What Does Water do for You?

Forms saliva (digestion)

Keeps mucosal membranes moist

Allows body's cells to grow, reproduce and survive

Flushes body waste, mainly in urine

Lubricates joints

Water is the major component of most body parts

Needed by the brain to manufacture hormones and neurotransmitters

Regulates body temperature (sweating and respiration)

Acts as a shock absorber for brain and spinal cord

Converts food to components needed for survival - digestion

Helps deliver oxygen all over the body

writes: "Even the hardiest bacteria need some moisture around them. They may survive complete dryness, but only in a dormant state, with all their processes arrested until they are reawakened by water".

Water carries intention and we are water based as humans. Making sure you have the healthiest water available to drink is also essential to optimizing your health and well being.

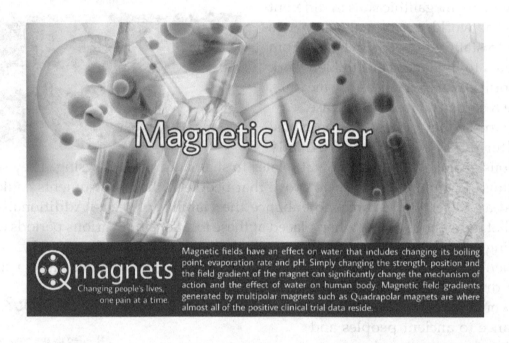

Magnetic fields have an effect on water that includes changing its boiling point, evaporation rate and pH. Simply changing the strength, position and the field gradient of the magnet can significantly change the mechanism of action and the effect of water on human body. Magnetic field gradients generated by multipolar magnets such as Quadrapolar magnets are where almost all of the positive clinical trial data reside.

Chapter 7

Complimentary Healing Resources

Nutrition. Supplements. Vitamins. Meditation. Creams. Lotions. Potions. Detox Food and much more. Healing powers of Medical Marijuana. Heavy Metal Detox Foods.

 (Full credit and my deepest appreciation to Ms. Tammy Nathan Horton for her critical contribution :)

Contrary to the common allopathic approach, in healing and health, a one size fits all solution is most often not the case. We are all as unique as our fingerprints and we all, at some time in our lives, need of a little help from our friends.

In this same approach Biomagnetism and its effects can be optimized and enhanced if an individual is plateauing in their convalescence. The methods discussed in this chapter will briefly outline some tools that can improve or promote further healing which can be used in addition to biomagnetism. Not every modality will suit the individual, but this chapter helps to explain the concepts of why and how it works with biomagnetism and where to look to research if it is something that is right for you.

As with all themes discussed in this book using applied kinesiology is always advised to see if a modality will best suit the situation and the individual at any given moment. Having a clear set of intentions, a connection to source and a specific question with a yes or no answer, is key for using our intuitive gifts. Muscle testing for a modality and usage or dose for parameters is always advised for all methods always. It truly is a wonderful tool to have to guide you on your road to health improvements. Once you get it will be like riding a bike - you never forget how to. It is quite amazing.

In the realm of vibrational modalities there are so many truly incredible and supportive tools one can use that come from nature for healing. We, being organic beings from the soil (soul) and of the salt (plasma), find we resonate best with using natures remedies in a slow and steady manner. We do not develop chronic illnesses overnight and we have to have that same understanding as we approach healing those conditions. There are rarely quick fixes, pills or potions. If someone claims this, it is wise to take caution. Slow and steady is always the best. Less is more. As above so below. We can anticipate the duration of our healing upward would correspond directly with our cascade to illness downward. In illness there is always health and we must realize and tap into this vibration within ourselves to ignite and catalyze further positive healing. No matter what level our healing needs to be experienced on, spiritual, mental or physical, we are a whole being and should treat our healing and experiences as such.

The stars shine brightest in the darkness. No matter if you are using biomagnetism therapy for a pulled tendon in your shoulder or to promote self-healing of a long battled chronic illness there is ALWAYS more room for more health, always. Even if they are only baby steps. When the body is treated as a perfect machine of health, given the right conditions, the body will always find homeostasis and thus find a will and a way to better health. The goal is always to allow the body to remember what balance is so that eventually it runs on its own like a fine-tuned race car on auto pilot. Let us explore some of the tools for optimization.

1. Breath Work

The saying "30 days without food, 3 days without water and 3 minutes without air ", puts our survival priorities in order of importance. Without proper oxygenation of our plasma our bodies are unable to complete the necessary conversion to create energy and sustain life. We often overlook the significant importance of the air we take in. It is an automatic process that we often don't think about unless we are ill with a lung infection or having a panic attack. But yogis say that the first body to get sick is the Pranic Body- the eighth etheric light body, the breath body. Traditional Chinese Medicine believes that wind at the neck is the first point of entry for illness. Just noticing the difference between the long and relaxed deep belly breath of a baby compared to the short shallow upper chest breaths of a stressed-out person says it all. If we can take one thing away from Wim Hof and Yogananda we can understand that prana is the most under-valued measurement of health and vitality as such should be given far more attention.

Experiment. When you awake in the new day place your left hand ring finger on the right nostril and left thump on left nostril. Use thumb and finger to open and close each nostril independently. Breathe ten breaths in through only left nostril, closing right nostril with finger, then reverse for ten breaths and repeat. You will notice each day you try this that one nostril (Sun or Moon) is more open than the other.

The Right nostril is the Yang or the Pingala channel which represents active, alert, awake and stimulated energetic status. (similar to the red magnet). If it is your left it is the opposite, yin, cooling, relaxed, tired, feminine, Ida channel (similar to black magnet properties and the left side of the body-moon). The most simple and effective pranayama to teach our children is called Nadi Shodna (alternate nostril breathing). To change the mental state from one to the other simply close the nostril of the side you would like to change - so want to become awake? Plug the left. Want to fall asleep? Plug the right. Long deep belly breathing for three minutes with that nostril closed. Like magic your dominant nostril will shift and so will your entire system.

There are many ways we can play with the pranic energy. The Mahabandha (the great lock) combined with the one-minute breath is said to cure ALL disease if mastered. Nauli kriya- the rolling of the belly combined with breath is also deeply healing. The main focus on all breathing is to breath into the belly, navel always moves first on the inhale, then the ribs then the clavicle, exhale is the reverse. Mantra is also helpful when the mind wanders. Singing is also beneficial for breathing. Remember that the lungs are not only the site for gas exchange, but also for detoxification. The deeper the breath the greater the exchange of molecules, gravity makes the blood in the lower lungs greater in volume, if we are breathing shallowly then we are not getting to the area that needs to detox. It is such an undervalued and simple solution to better health. Try set a reminder each hour perhaps to do long deep breathing for three minutes. Exercise. Sing. Move. Prana is more important than we realize. For more exercises the book Prana, Pranee, Pranayam by Yogi Bhajan has many great exercises.

The science is there it is up to us to do the work to enhance our healing abilities naturally and effectively with beauty and simplicity just as nature intended.

https://www.wimhofmethod.com

https://www.amazon.com/Praana-Praanee-Pranayam-Exploring-Technology-ebook/dp/B00MO3GNGG

2. Healthy Water

How amazing is water? It defies the laws of science, expanding in cold, contracting in the heat, taking four shapes- liquid, gas, solid and net matrix. It composes 70-80 percent of our cellular makeup. It has a memory. It can change shape based on our thoughts alone (see Emoto Water Study). Communities living in blue

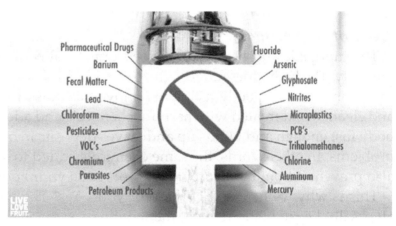

zones have had access to glacial hexagonal shaped water springs which have been associated with their longevity. Natures fauna always chooses moving water over still ponds. Why? Magnetized and energized water does exactly that to our systems. But it has to be the right kind of water. Tap water and bottled water are loaded with things like chloramines, chlorine, fluoride, spores, cysts, hormones, bacteria and metals depending on geographical location. It is of utmost importance to drink clean and pure living water. Pure water can cause water poisoning in cases of dehydration (reverse osmosis- dead water) as well as cold water can kill a horse- room temperature or warm is best always not to shock the system.

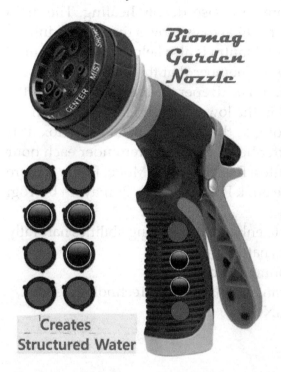

Biomag Garden Nozzle

Creates Structured Water

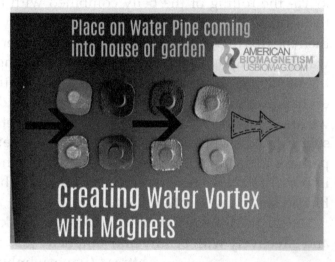

Place on Water Pipe coming into house or garden

AMERICAN BIOMAGNETISM USBIOMAG.COM

Creating Water Vortex with Magnets

Dr. Garcia's friend developed a simple structured water magnet arrangement that I sell at biomaghealer.com or you can make one on your own with magnets. We also sell biomag structured water garden nozzles.

SALT of the Earth and Sea?

The inorganic and heavily processed unnatural compounded salt is actually toxic to the body. The body does not recognize or need this compound and thus causes high fluid retention due to the body trying to remove this poison. It has been chemically bleached and cleaned and treated with harmful chemicals and additives. It has no way to clear the body fast enough and builds up and leaves deposits in organs and tissue, causing health problems. In other words, the same chemicals added to salt to prevent water absorption also prevent it from being properly absorbed in your body.

This is why we hear salt is "bad for you". Yes! The wrong salt is, absolutely. Shortly after salty began being refined, mental illness statistically increased. It should be noted that what do doctors give to patients to help regulate manic-depressive patients? Lithium, a trace mineral in natural salt that has been removed and is missing from table salt. The right salt is freshly harvested natural and unrefined sea salt, it is loaded with minerals that our body recognizes and needs and craves. The best natural salts come straight from the sea in origin. The best are Himalayan Sea Salt (be cautious of fake dyed salts), Real Salt brand, Celtic Sea Salt brand and Jacobsen Sea Salt Company. Make sure you do your research and trust your source as with anything.

Salt is most effective in stabilizing irregular heart rhythms, vital to the extraction of excess acidity from the cells in the body, particularly neurons, it regulates blood sugar, it is vital for the generation of hydroelectric energy in the body. It facilitates neural signaling for communication and information processing from brain to fingertip and back, it is vital for the absorption of food particles in the GI tract, clears the lungs of mucus and sticky phlegm, clears catarrh and congestion from the sinuses, is a strong natural antihistamine, anti-viral, anti-parasitic and anti-bacterial, prevents muscle cramps, is vital for sleep regulation and circadian rhythms, is vital for saliva production, is vital for bone structure formation and making bones firm (osteoporosis is a result of salt and water shortage). It is vital for the prevention of gout and arthritis, maintains sexual libido, prevents varicose veins, reduces double chin, and it contains 80 mineral elements that the body needs for life sustaining functions. Bad salt does the exact opposite.

Unrefined salt is real salt and it synonymous with life today as we know it as well as billions of years ago. Lack of adequate salt lends to dehydration, birth defects, organ failure, decay, diseases, premature aging, and premature death. The problem with salt is that beginning in 1923 processors began kiln drying salt at high temperatures above 1200F'. These extreme temperatures cause alterations to its chemical structure. Not only does heat ruin its original natural form but during the refining process 82 out of 84 essential minerals are removed, leaving only inorganic sodium chloride. Table salt becomes basically an inorganic sodium compound to which "anti-caking" additives have been added such as aluminum hydroxide, silica aluminate, sodium ferrocyanide, tai-calcium phosphate, stearic acid and others. Aluminum has been implicated in Alzheimers and dementia and is very difficult to remove from the brain once it enters the blood brain barrier.

As a side note Himalayan Salt caves give off beneficial negative ions just like black magnets. Salt lamps are a beautiful addition to any room and have been proven to reduce allergies due to their antihistamine properties. Salt Rocks!!!

Baking Soda

For instant healing benefits for acid states, if needed, use baking soda 1/4 tsp added to warm water instantly alkalizes the body, increases VO2max, cardiac performance and reduces lactic acid.

Remember this one thing. We must always change the water in the fish tank, right? Otherwise it gets dingy, smelly and toxic. In the same way we need to change our water environment, but it has to be the right environment. We need to replace our plasma with plasma. Low salt diets are detrimental to health, the right salt diet adds vitality and electricity to our systems and

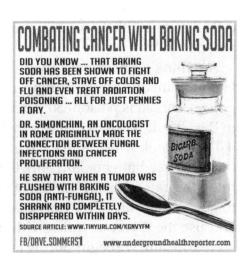

enables our cellular reactions to take place for the best health we can attain. Salt is life, water is life, oxygen is life- the right kinds of these molecules make or break your vitality and energetic potential.

3. Nutrition ~ Let Food by Thy Medicine and Medicine by Thy Food

Let us focus on macro elements now that we understand the importance of clean micro-nutrients. Our food. We are what we eat and food is our medicine.

Food should be called our medicine and we would see and choose much differently. We are the only species on the plane-t that doesn't know what to eat, have you ever stopped to consider this fact? We have hundreds of thousands of "diet" books and yet everyone is still utterly confused. This is by design. The food pyramid is wrong!!!

We do not require three square meals of 80 percent grains per day. This is not how our ancestors ate and it is why we have a world full of unhealthy and obese humans. When we shop the middle of the grocery aisles we are asking for trouble. Things that have more than 5 ingredients or an expiration date longer than three days are a NO NO.

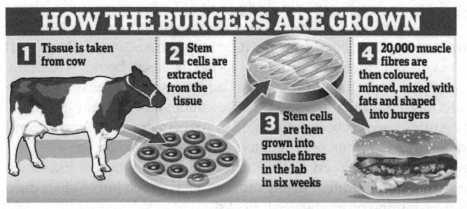

Anything with a preservative should be thrown out- it is poison. Anything injected with antibiotics and hormones should be avoided as well as anything sprayed with roundup or chemicals or soaked in ozone for 30 minutes or peroxide and water. Impossible burgers are cloned replicating cells that cost little to manufacture and use artificial lab ingredients untested for health and nutrition.

Anything with artificial dyes like blue lake or red lake should also be avoided. Sugar, HFCS, palm oil, canola, safflower, anything bleached, etc. should be tossed!!! Rapeseed is poison, canola is poison- 80 percent of Whole Foods items are coated in canola. (banned in the UK). It is cheap that is why it is used but highly unstable with heat and very toxic.

Do not cook with oils that have a low smoke point. Cook with high heat oils like coconut or sunflower, butter or lard only. Oils that are solid at room temperature. All others convert into trans fats with application of heat. If you decide to eat legumes or grains always soak to get rid of lectins, they can cause leaky gut. Use a variety of cooked and raw vegetables and use the glycemic index with all foods to regulate glucose response. The minute we secrete insulin we begin storing fat. 90/10 rule- 90 percent healthful choices and 10 percent pleasure foods. Generally speaking, we are omnivores, we are not designed to digest cellulose, we do not have seven stomachs to make cud, we have sharp incisors as well as flat molars. We have a need for cobalamin (B12- cobalt) which we cannot obtain through vegan diets. Morally and ethically speaking veganism is the best - it allows us to eat the energy of the living plant and promote our own cellular electricity.

But even plants make their own chemical defenses such as calcium oxalate (kidney stones), phytates, saponins, terpenoids and more that can cause harm to our health if we don't know how to soak, cook or process them properly. Dose matters most with anything. Studies show that native tribes that consumed no grains (seeds of grasses) had no incidence of mental illness as well as dental cavities (Weston A Price, Linus Pauling) See Dr. William Davis' work at www.wheatbellyblog.com.

We are meant to eat a small amount of animal protein and fat but it is to be done with honor and reverence as the natives waste nothing, Kosher Noah Hide laws send up sparks for the soul. In this way we can honor the sacrifice for our own survival. "Our great mother does not take sides; she protects the balance of life. "Avatar. "Na'vi kill prayer- "I see you, brother and I thank you. Your spirit will go with Eywa, but your body stays behind to become part of the people".

We have become so disconnected from nature, our soil, our land, the place we come from. We are the earth, the salt of the earth. Born from the ashes to return again. We must look at food as a gift, a medicine and a blessing. Nothing should be wasted, rverything to be shared. A lot can be learned of a person by watching the way they eat. How they begin, their pace, their gratitude. Remember food contains water, water contains memory. The energy you put into your food imprints on every molecule. Vitamin L is most important of all. Vitamin Love. No one food is right for everyone. It is all trial and error. What Is good for you today may not be tomorrow. We have two powerful tools to use for our food intake, Our fingers to muscle test and our noses. Just because a food may smell amazing at first, the first scent of it will either feel good or not in your belly and intuition. Use these tools always. Even with supplements. You will be surprised how accurate they are.

Some beautiful books to read, *The Primal Blueprint* by Mark Sisson, *Nourishing Traditions* by Sally Fallon, *Nutrition and Physical Degeneration* by Weston A Price, Wheat Belly Dr William Davis, *Superfoods* by David Wolfe, *Spiritual Nutrition* by Gabriel Cousens. www.integrativenutrition.com

Pet Food

(if you love your pets don't feed them cereal (kibble) feed them your leftovers- feed them what they would eat in nature) DO NOT FEED PETS GRAINS EVER!!! Never ever feed Carnivorous cats grains- please read labels diligently. Grains cause chronic UTI's in felines and much worse. Look at your domesticated pet as a wild animal and feed them accordingly just like humans. See www.perfectlyrawsome.com for feeding calculators and proper pet nutrition. Always make sure to include raw meaty bones for dental health as well as essential fats for coat, brain and joints. Pets dont need to eat raw if you are not comfortable but you can easily feed them cooked human proteins at the same price as kibble. Pets will always go to the food they like the best so its good to sample a few choices to know what they like. For example, a bite size of cooked bison, beef, salmon, turkey and lamb. Each pet is different,but they do tell us right away what they like.

5. Sofleggio Music ~ Like Heals Like

Rules of Homeopathy

What is music? Sound waves of frequency and vibration that are mathematically combined to produce beauty of form, harmony and expression of emotion. Sound therapy is using frequency and vibration and intention to elicit a specific healing effect on an individual such as relaxation, chakra clearing or tuning of the entire etheric system. The ideal frequencies are solfeggio frequencies which complete the Fibonacci form or the sacred geometry of our light bodies. Each light body has a specific tone and a planetary energy that we can tap into using live musical instruments which are tuned to affect a specific healing benefit. For example, our first chakra the muladarha (root) is the color red and matches the frequency 396 Hertz and the planet Mars. This chakra when balanced liberates fear, guilt and trauma. When we have a soul who is communicating these emotions we can apply music that vibrates the same for 20 minutes with say a planetary gong and then always elevate one level for another 20 minutes- which would be 417 Hz on the scale. If a soul is expressing fear, lack of creativity, hesitance to change and the undoing of situations then we would apply 417 Hz for 20 minutes and follow with 528Hz to elevate.

- **Ut - 396 Hz** - turning grief into joy, liberating guilt and fear
- **Re - 417 Hz** - undoing situations and facilitating change
- **Mi - 528 Hz** - transformation and miracles (DNA repair)
- **Fa - 639 Hz** - reconnecting and balancing relationships
- **Sol - 741 Hz** - solving problems, expressions/solutions
- **La - 852 Hz** - awakening intuition, returning to spiritual order

If they present with brain fog, low self-esteem, turmoil, lack of self-worth, hatred and depression we would apply 528 Hz then elevate to 639Hz. If they present difficulty opening up, matters of the heart, disharmony, sadness and relationship issues we would apply 639Hz and elevate to 741 Hz. If they are presenting with many problems and no solutions, issues communicating, people not hearing them when they speak and throat issues we would apply 741 Hz and follow with 852Hz. If they are unbalanced, heavy, feeling lack of inspiration, lack of divine connection especially to their soul we would apply 852 Hz and follow with 963Hz. If they are demonstrating hardship in feeling connected and having doubts, not seeing the whole picture we would apply 963Hz and then 1074Hz.

We can use a simple app for tuning or we can use a mini frequency generator or a gong, tuning forks, chimes, copper plates, crystal or metal singing bowls or any instrument that is tuned to these particular frequencies. While applying magnet therapy the sound waves will enhance the healing. We can also fine tune our therapies by using particular frequencies that match our organ systems. Remember each biomagnetic pair has its own frequency and when sound is applied it only improves and speeds the benefits.

Lumimaries, Sounds, Colors and Metres

The following is a table of the audio frequencies, colors and meters analogous to the planetary (luminary) cycles in the order of the octaves. Click on a name of a cycles (first column) to read the individual description.

Explanation:

Cycle: Duration of the period in days or years frequency: The tuning forks are tuned in this frequencies

Hertz: Number of cycles per second octave: The number of octaves is based on the period.tone: The designations of the tones.a1: The frequency of the corresponding chromatic a1diff. 440 Hz: The difference to 440 Hz, given in cents.

Color: The color corresponding to the duration of the period in order of the octaves. BPM: beats per minute pendulum: A pendulum of the given length (in centimeters) swings with the frequency given in the same row (in bpm). It can be used as a time reference; in case a metronome is not available.

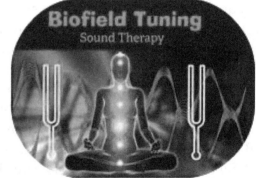

Ideally all resonant frequencies would be intentionally created within an electromagnetic field to produce enhanced energetic tones. These tones should be tuned to 432Hz and not 440Hz (like our current radio music which is proven to cause feelings of chaos and anger) All of these tones are in alignment with PHI or the golden ratio - aka the Fibonacci number sequence.

There is much debate around the 432 versus 440 tuning. The story behind the deception can easily be researched on the link below. The bottom line is there are corresponding sounds and tones that can be applied to the biofield whilst in a biomagnetism session. It can be as simple as playing beautiful spa like music, binaural beats, solfeggio tones, theta or gamma electronically generated music to as complex as live sound therapy using instruments that are tailored to the organ systems and emotions that require the healing.

As long as the music is aligned with the soul the healing will be enhanced. One caveat and a very important one. Some traumas can be brought up by certain frequencies that the client is not ready to deal with. For example, gongs can bring up PTSD for war veterans. In a case such as this it would be ideal to cease that instrument or music and find something they choose. Or no music at all until the client has settled back into a relaxed state. We heal in many layers and we heal cyclically. Certain organs also hold onto certain emotions as well. Psychosomatic healing can be deep and very, very, healing but the client has to be ready to venture into those places to promote that healing also. Prana and emotions coincide always. Just always watch your client and be very in tune and sensitive to their breathing patterns to gauge what is needed in a given moment. Better to know and be prepared for anything that may arise. The beauty of music is that 99 percent of the time it will create a gorgeous experience for healing for both the healer and the client alike.

Some beautiful reading material and resources:

The Cosmic Octave by: Cousteau

The Musical Theory of Existence by: Steve Madison

https://meinlsonicenergy.com/en/home

https://iesoundtherapy.com

https://earthpulse.net/pythagorean-pemf-432-hz-528-tuning/

5. The Royal Rife Machine

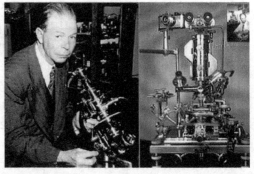

On the theme of frequency and vibration there is an amazing healing device that was invented in the 1920's by a scientist named Royal Rife. These healing machines are able to shatter organisms using frequencies similar to an opera singer shattering a glass with the perfect pitch. In nature everything has its own radio station and when we tune into the perfect dialed in station, we get a clear crisp sound. In that same way when we dial into the frequency of an organism, we can kill it quickly and easily the key is knowing which frequency to apply. For this we muscle test!!!! There are many great documentaries on Royal Rife and his BX BY cancer research. A search engine " Rife killing under microscope" can demonstrate the many amazing powers of a rife. They are labeled as quackery however aren't many things that work? The proof is in the product and the evidence firsthand.

There are many great rife machines out there at many different price ranges and functionalities here is a list from least to greatest:

1. The most affordable is a free a simple tone generator. It is a sine wave general tone. You can use it to program crystals or clear your home like you would burning sage. It is a great beginner resource. Now this is not the best because the strength of the frequency is very weak but it can still be useful for many applications.

www.onlinetonegenerator.com

2. Mini tone generator- this is a mini device that can be used with any orgone piece simply connected with a wire to amplify a given space- www.akaida.com makes some beautiful ones. But the generator you can find its called FG085 mini multi tone generator.

> https://www.fruugo.us/jyetech-fg085-minidds-function-generator-with-panel/p-52180072-105043027?language=en&ac=g oogle&gclid=Cj0KCQjwrsGCBhD1ARIsALILBYp8UKtKKfiVaqwe NQBM48uZ4Niqaa-_tOIAUObS8cHX1zNWkvXEnT4aAhW3EALw_wcB

3. Hulda Clark Zapper- great and basic for contact mode only-https://drclarkstore.com/dr-clark-zapper-syncrozap-with-wristbands-model-a11/

4. Spooky2- the cheapest generator with the most functionality- has PEMF, Scalar, Tens, Plasma, contact, remote (quantum), biofeedback scans and so much more, the best library of all rife programs on the market. However, it is glitchy and tricky if you are not tech savvy. https://www.spooky2-mall.com

5. BCX Ultra- a very good basic rife machine, has great bulbs, foot bath and plasma for a big room, all of Rife's original frequencies. Limited programs, very basic great for plug and play- not technical as compared to others, no biofeedback scans. https://www.hymbas.com/bcx-ultra-rife-machine-all-products.php?_vsrefdom=adwords&gclid=Cj0KCQjwrsGCBhD1ARIsALILBYrqBjA6qoBo_qHehMuW2sLcm8D9XfJUyXKuYBLfbIVu6rxVi2OuHAwaAqLsEALw_wcB

6. GB-4000 Mopa- This guy is HUGE! In price and size and sound. Has all of the Original frequencies but not many other applications, many report being fully cured with the GB due to its powerful output. https://www.thegb4000.com/Frequency-Machine/M.O.P.A-Amplifier

7. Pearl -M Resonant light- This rife is amplifier only like the GB but has the power to do a larger area, it is very attractive looking and has amazing reviews. https://www.resonantlight.ca

8. True Rife- By far this is the best rife available- It has many applications such as Ozone bulb, GRS scan for biofeedback, contact mode, overnight bulb during sleep, q-2 bulb (strongest on the market), spiral bulb, grounding bed sheet, colloidal silver maker, foot bath, Halo crystal coated bulb and now the q-5 bulb which is the most powerful to date. The true rife has many many cure cases a fantastic customer support group and a certification program for practitioners. It is the Ferrari of Rife machines but it is very expensive. Well worth it if you are looking to heal. www.truerife.com

Contrary to some beliefs a rife machine is NOT a healing machine. It will not repair damaged cells or put DNA proteins back together as some programs on some rife machines say. It is a pathogen killing machine and it does so very very very well when the perfect frequency is found and applied for the proper duration at the proper wave form. There is a post protocol for any rife treatment and that is detox.

When many microscopic organisms have their cell walls obliterated there is a die off reaction (herxheimer) and one can feel quite sick after wards - flulike symptoms are normal, hydration is needed as is proper rest and nutrition. Most herxheimers last a day, sometimes it does not occur. But if you are hitting the nail on the head there usually is a die off reaction so be prepared to give yourself some TLC. Over time the sessions should get easier to tolerate. Do not rife more than every other day for long periods. Like anything Less is more when it comes to Mother Nature. Be wise, in tune to your needs and always muscle test it.

www.youtube.com/watch?v=rHJXBLuqh60

6. Homeopathy

Greek homoiopathes meant "having like feelings or affections, sympathetic."

Homeopathy is the "treatment of disease by medicines (usually in minute doses) that in a healthy person would produce symptoms like those of the disease" [1].

The American Institute of Homeopathy was formed in 1844.

At the time, homeopathy was widely used in the US, both by doctors and in the home, and only reached its peak of popularity in the 1870s. At the turn of the 19th century, there were more homeopathic hospitals in the US than any other kind.

Allopathy is the "curing of disease by inducing an action of a different kind (to homeopathy)" [1]. The American Medical Association (AMA) (of doctors) was formed in 1847 to promote surgery and (non-homeopathic) medicine, and specifically aimed to overcome homeopathy in the US.

A member of the AMA could be struck off for consulting or even being married to a homeopathic physician. Other therapies such as electrotherapy - also popular - were not targeted in the same way at that time – the Flexner report debunking "non-scientific medicine" did not appear until 1910 [9].

Homeopathy was developed in the 18th century by a German doctor by the name of Samuel Hahnemann, who founded a system based on the ancient concept that " like cures like". It is based on the idea that large doses of a substance will cause a symptom, while very small doses of that same substance will cure it. Scientifically it has not yet been explained how homeopathy works, but new theories in quantum physics are shedding light on the process, even though it has been highly suppressed and under researched. And for good reason. It costs pennies for a remedy as compared to patented allopathic pharmaceuticals. Therefore, there is no profitability for the corporations.

What we do know is that a carefully selected homeopathic remedy acts as a trigger to the body's healing processes. This concept is the forerunner of vaccines in modern times. However, the difference is night and day in terms of a substance, to where it is the "energetic trace or imprint" or frequency of an item which makes it far safer, yet very effective. It is very popular to this day in India and used and widely promoted. However, many single remedies are now being removed from shelves in North America- because it works!

Homeopathic remedies range from flora to fauna to minerals (cell salts) and even to diseased tissue called "nosodes". Nosodes, are a very special type of remedy for special types of cases. But remember that it is not the diseased tissue itself, but it is the energetic vibrational imprint of the disease. It may sound repulsive at first but if you can see it in a way of energy and not material it makes a lot of sense. Like cancels out like.

Everything is neutralized and healing is restored. Often times, the homeopath will consult the client to get to know certain quirks and behaviors I test for particular remedies. Say a client comes in expressing a busy and very organized life style, wearing bright colors and having an aversion to rain and an affinity for fresh flowers in her home(we call these miasms- symptoms or expressions) we could perhaps look into a bee remedy called-Apis. This remedy could also be used for acute symptoms also such as an insect bite or a swollen eyelid on your dog. In the same action the bee venom swells, reddens and irritates the area we would choose Apis for this also.

Homeopathic remedies can used for behaviors, emotions, addictions, spiritual sickness, and diseases and they can be made from ANYTHING! And they are the vibrational signature of that substance. They are dilutions of the original substance that are shaken and diluted so many times that only the energy remains. Remember water has a memory. Homeopathic remedies are always made in a liquid medium. For this reason. The lower the number of potencies, the more physical the issue it addresses, the higher the number the more etheric. Homeopathy can be used in many mediums such as pellets, drops, creams, and gels- but always in a water base. They are very simple to make with a radionics machine. Books can be found on Ebay such as Hahnemann, Kent, Boericke materia medica but new prints are rare.

It is impossible to get a true homeopathic remedy maker; they have been banned or burned. There are a few out there but for now the best we have are electronic versions called radionics machines. Some great ones are BERKANA Labs boards that attach to spooky 2 rife if you have one. They are just amazing and always sold out. www.berkanalabs. com They also provide a great user manual that is very very useful. The other product that is great are Bionetix machines on Ebay out of the UK. They are the only company providing these machines of quality and proof of work https://www.ebay.com/usr/bionetix?_trksid=p2047675.l2559 but also not inexpensive. Limits are endless for vibrational healing. If you are looking for more information on homeopathy the Canadian College of Homeopathics has many great resources. https://ochm.ca

I also greatly recommend Bach Flower Essences for the highest form of healing energetically. There is nothing more powerful than the bloom energy of a flower. Bach found that in all of his homeopathic research there were no greater healings than that he witnessed with Flower Remedies. They are absolutely fantastic and immediate. Having a 100 remedy kit from Helios Homeopathy is amazing to have on hand for your tool kit. (See "*Vibrational Medicine*" by Richard Gerber)

Remedies can also be made without a copier using the old methods of dilution and shaking. One only needs to research and you will find how.

Some great companies to purchase your remedies:

www.boiron.com

www.hylands.com

www.helios.co.uk

www.bachflower.com

7. Meditation ~ No Place Like Om

Ahhhhh to be zen! Ommmmmm. Ohnnnnnnng. Yaaaaaaaaammmmmm ~ Whatever mantra you choose it replaces the monkey chatter (vrittis) with a much sweeter and much more serene mind (man) song/tune(tra) rather than the constant jumping of thoughts. It is a common misconception that meditation is meant to be zen and peaceful.

The purpose of meditation is to bring the stuff up to the surface to be healed from the layers of consciousness- emotional, subconscious, collective unconscious, ancestral layers. It is to be able to notice the thoughts as they come up and return your mind to the focus rather than getting lost in the story. It's like taking the hand of the toddler and gently bringing them back to sit at a table to do a task. The toddler will keep trying to go do something else just like the thoughts will keep distracting the meditation. Each time to take their hand once again and guide them back to the table. In the same way one guides their mind back to the meditation task and not the story or the fantasy being created to distract. It takes many hours of practice to get to know the space where the mind meets the heart and soul. When we are born, we should learn this and breath work first. It would save a lot of time later in life.

It is easier to build strong children than to repair broken adults. Meditation does this and more. Yogis recommend beginning with a 40 day meditation as it takes 40 days to break a habit. 90 days to create a new habit. 120 days to confirm a habit and 1000 days to master a habit so that it becomes you. A habit is a subconscious chain reaction between the mind, the glandular system and the nervous system.

We develop habits at a very young age. Some serve our highest destiny and some do not. Meditation can help you develop new and deeply ingrained habits that serve your highest potential.

In Tibet most of the statues of Buddha's are positions of quiet, inward contemplation. "Know Thyself to Be True" was inscribed over the Oracle of Delphi where ancient Greeks would go for universal knowing.

There are many ways to meditate. There are many books on meditation. When starting out its best to have small victories. There is always time for a 3-minute meditation, get the app Insight Timer and meditate with others, or find a guided meditation on YouTube there are so many. Find the right voice that soothes you and you can have some pretty powerful experiences. Kundalini yoga meditations are very, very powerful as well. Some great teachers are Catalyst Yogi or Karena Virginia, Sadhguru or Meditative Mind. There are so many kinds you just have to find what is right for you but the amazing

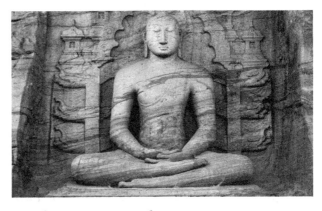

healing benefits are countless. Some meditations have mantras, chants or songs, some are only breath alone, some involve counting and other visualizations. All of which help you go deeper into your personality, your heart, your soul, your shadow, your higher self and your purpose. What better gift than to give yourself the ability to know and love yourself. This combined with a biomagnetism session could be very very powerful indeed. Meditation with magnets is like amped up soul work. Give it a try you might love what you find.

www.3HO.org
www.insighttimer.com
www.libraryofteachings.org

8. Pulsed Electro Magnetic Field ~ PEMF

Pulsed Electro Magnetic Field healing is similar to BiomagHealing only but using electricity application that creates a pulsed magnet field at a range of Gauss versus magnetism. It has been proven in studies to have benefits for pain reduction and significant benefits for preventing rouleax in the blood - the abnormal clumping of blood cells. As well as benefits to speed healing of bone fractures (FDA approved for this purpose). It is currently used by numerous equine veterinarians with much success. It can improve athletic performance, reduce inflammation, stimulate cell metabolism, aid in speed of recover and increase cellular oxygen uptake by 200 percent. Thus reducing pain associated with lack of sufficient oxygen. Isn't this the root of all dis-ease- the lack of oxygen and an acidic state? Why of course. Wonder why research on static magnet application has not been studied deeper...things that make you go hmmmm? For more resources on PEMF visit www.drpawluk.com or read the book

Healing is Voltage by Dr. Jerry Tennant. There are a wide variety of devices that can be used for small or large field of work. Earth Pulse is a wonderful moderate version with up to 2000 Gauss (adjustable and programable) and wonderful sleep and repair programs. Higher pulsed machines that go up into the 10,000s should be used with caution as they are not natural forms from nature (those with pacemakers, stents, pumps, hardware implants and soft implants, pregnancy, chemotherapy patients are contraindicated). The body knows best what Mother Nature intended anything other should be used with research and precaution. PEMF therapy can be beneficial but biomagnetism makes for a better therapy due to its lack of 60Hz plug in the wall. Nature is always best and always first. PEMF machines can be great for short term use and application but it is not portable and does not make sense long term. Some great devices are the PEMF 120, Bemer, Earth Pulse, Teslafit, and the Hugo. There are also PEMF mats that have crystals and infrared imbedded. Again, muscle test and read read read up to find what is best for your needs. Pay attention to Gauss, programs, accessories and range of field. Dr Pawluk has a great comparison chart on his site as well.

A great intro book is called *PEMF-the Fifth Element of Health* by Bryant A Meyers

Healing is Voltage Dr Jerry Tennant

www.drpawluk.com

www.us.hugopemf.com

www.pemf120.com

www.earthpulse.net

https://life.bemergroup.com

www.teslafit.comn order to properly select a remedy. There is an intimate process to selecting, dowsing, or muscle.

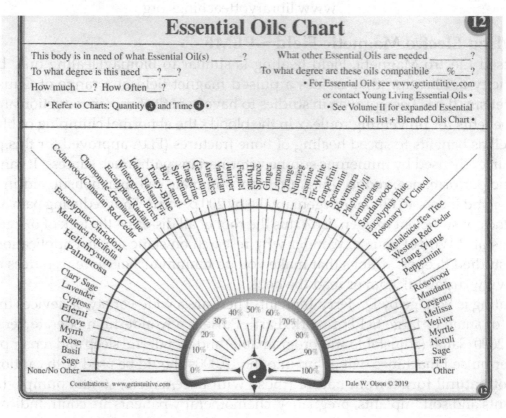

9. Essential Oils

Essential oils and aromatherapy have gained a lot of popularity in recent years. Their powerful healing abilities have really come into the mainstream and for good reason. Essential oils have been used for many centuries, the first documented being the oil of the cardamom pod over 5000 years ago. Many precious plant-based oils have been used in ceremonies like burials in Egypt with myrrh, cinnamon, frankincense, and coriander. The three wise men brought these gifts to Jesus. We have seen their use and benefits in apothecaries and medicine cabinets from past to present time. Oils are essentially the sunlight, the soil, the water, the air and the minerals and the energy during their entire growth cycle. That's why the energy in creating the oil is so very important to consider when using or purchasing a particular brand.

Oils are made from the bark, seeds, roots, resins, fruit, skins, stems, flowers, threads and leaves of plants which are prepared, extracted and distilled into its pure oil-based form. Oils are classified according to their notes. Base, middle and top notes. Base notes last the longest in fragrance about 8 hours whereas middle last 2-4 hours and top the least in duration 1-2 hours. When combined a base can make a middle or top last longer. Oils can also be categorized by frequency in Mega Hertz as well.

When we use a particular oil which is diluted always in a carrier oil we can increase the overall healing frequency or use that oil to uplift a given individual or healing session. We can also diffuse the oil in a diffuser or put a few drops in hot water so that it permeates the room. There are some oils that are not for skin use, many herb oils are also not allowed for children or during pregnancy due to their powerful properties such as sage for example will induce labor. Eucalyptus radiata is not to be used with children but eucalyptus globulus is okay to use. Citrus oils are skin irritants and even when diluted can harm the skin and cause acid burns.

Therefore, it is very important to always research and be sure before using. Oils that are safe are called GRAS (generally regarded as safe). There are also oils that can be used Neat- undiluted such as lavender on a burn. But there aren't many that can be used Neat. Some companies even test so pure that they can be used internally with proper guidance with a trained practitioner. Raindrop chakra therapy can also be extremely therapeutic.

Below demonstrates the elevating frequencies of oils. Bulgarian Rose Oil used to have the highest frequency at 320MHz but recently has taken a second place to Idaho Blue Spruce at 428 MHz.

The Science ~ the Rose Frequency

In 1992, Bruce Tainio of Tainio Technology, a division of Eastern Washington State University, Cheney, WA, developed equipment to measure electrical frequency in humans and foods. This equipment was used in a research study at Johns Hopkins University to determine the relationships between frequency and diseases. Results from the studies:

While holding a cup of coffee, one participant's frequency dropped from 66 MHz to 58 MHz (-8 MHz). Another participant drank the coffee, his frequency dropped from 66 MHz to 52 MHz (-14 MHz). After inhaling an essential oil of 75 MHz or higher, their frequency returned to normal in less than one minute.

While holding a cigarette another subject's frequency dropped from 65 MHz to 48 MHz (-17 MHz); smoking the cigarette, his frequency dropped to 42 MHz (-23 MHz), the *same frequency as cancer.*

Essential oils in the higher frequency ranges tend to influence the emotions.

Essential oils in the lower frequencies have more effect on structural and physical changes, including cells, hormones, and bones, as well as viruses, bacteria, and fungi. Similarly, to the potencies of homeopathic remedies.

Essential oils do not resonate with the toxins in our bodies.

This incompatibility is what helps eliminate the toxins from our systems.

Essential oils also do not resonate with negative emotions.

Allowing us a greater opportunity to release them.

Best Companies to buy from:

https://www.doterra.com/US/en
http://originalswissaromatics.com
https://www.youngliving.com
https://www.sunrosearomatics.com
https://mountainroseherbs.com

Addiction/Detox	53a	Bacteria. Viral
Addiction/Detox	66b	Nervous Tics. Facial Paralysis
Addiction/Detox	51a	Snorting Drugs. Nasal. Nose2x
Addiction/Detox	88b	Smokers. Shortness of Breath
Addiction/Detox	126b	Smoking. Birth control. Obesity
Addiction/Detox	105b	GI Discomfort
Addiction/Detox	106a	Pancreas Body -Pancreas Tail
Addiction/Detox	59a	Alcohol. Drugs.
Addiction/Detox	170b**	Alcohol. Buzz Kill.Kidney .gout

10. Detox

Dr. Garcia's placement pages for Detox and Addiction

"It's a dirty job but someone's gotta do it." When we enter into the realm of healing we often focus on the end goal, the feeling of optimal health and happiness. Which in itself is very important and absolutely necessary. Being able to visualize yourself living in the end goal, living the dream so to speak is the key to success in any goal setting. However, we often neglect the housekeeping needed to maintain our path to that goal. Let's talk about plumbing for a quick moment. If all of our anatomy is composed of vessels and capillaries and tubes, then wouldn't we want to make sure that those pathways are wide open and clear of congestion? Who wants to sit in a traffic jam when we could cruise on an open road? In that same way we need to ensure that there is no mucus, phlegm, stool, calcified stones, clotted blood, adhesion or obstruction. How do we do this? We must learn how to clean and clear our vessels and excretory pathways in order to ensure a long and fruitful lifetime of use.

Let's start from the outside, our largest organ, our skin. The only way to detox hormone disruptors from plastics and dryer sheets is by sweating. How do we do this? Exercise and FAR-infared sauna. Sweating 30 minutes most days of the week purifies the sweat glands and detoxifies the skin. It is the ONLY way to detox phthalates (PVC plastics)

Respiratory system/ circulatory system- we detox the heart and lungs with exercise, deep breathing, and hydrotherapy (Ishnaan/Wim Hof method/Post Athletic Ice Baths). Ice cold water promotes the flushing of all capillaries and reduces inflammatory responses, in every extremity of even the smallest size. Yogis knew if the student performed cold showers prior to meditation due to the size of their auras. If the aura was small the student did not have a cold shower. Ishnaan is performed in the morning prior to sadhana. The entire body is vigorously rubbed to warmth in the cold water using circular massage strokes, paying particular attention to the vital organs and glands for about 5 whole minutes. They believed that hot showers chased the illness inward, so hot baths were to be taken for relaxation purposes. Showers were to be taken cold. But never on the third eye area for this is a remedy for insomnia. Three minutes of ice cold water on the third eye will rid insomnia. Heat on the head will calm excessive emotions.

Renal system is where we get serious now. The kidneys filter all of our water. This is the site of all detox that is critical to support health and vitality. If we have stones in our kidneys we will have chronic UTI's which leads to bacterial overgrowth and then bladder and kidney diseases (get some D mannose/ kidney tea and cranactin at the first signs of tugging/pain). If we have calcifications from high oxalic acid from things like spinach, or minerals from soda, refined and processed grains our body will make stones in the kidneys as well as cause things like erectile dysfunction and bladder control problems. We must do a kidney cleanse annually at least. Hulda clark kidney cleanse is simple and easy and effective. In addition, using parsley, celery, hydrangea, ginger, cranberry and black cherry are very beneficial to include in your diet. Marshmallow and gravel root tea dissolves calculi as well as chanca piedra (aka stone breaker). There are many supportive herbs for the kidneys. But proper diet and exercise there is really no substitute in that matter.

There is an amazing book called" *It's the Liver Stupid*" by James Robert Clark that can be eye opening as to how many symptoms can connect to a liver problem. Everything from bowling ball syndrome to food allergies. The liver filters all of our blood, processes all drugs, chemicals, food macronutrients, minerals, vitamins and makes all of our hormones and cholesterol. There is really no other organ that performs so many functions per day. The liver also encapsulates toxins in a protective cholesterol shell (gallstone) when necessary, when the stones grow larger, they are moved into the gallbladder for storage permanently. For life! With proper bile production the stones will be processed through the intestines and excreted. But for many who are facing chronic illness, our food supply is so lacking in nutrients to make proper amounts of bile (taurine and glycine are precursors) that the stones just sit in storage. Over time the contents of the stones can produce many symptoms such as Irritable Bowel, food allergies, depression, Gerd, high blood pressure, frozen shoulder, arthritis, gout, allergies and more. The Hulda Clark liver cleanse is not easy but well worth it. The book by Andreas Mortiz called the "*Miracle gallbladder and liver cleanse*" does what it claims, if followed step by step. Pay careful attention to the TCM organ clock times and eating only carbs if you chose to eat on the cleanse day. More stones are expelled if wet fasting is done. It is a pretty amazing detox that really gives so much renewal to your health and vitality.

If purging stones or disintegrating calculi isn't for you at the moment, there are other milder forms of binding toxins things like zeolites, French green and bentonite clays, diatomaceous earth, msm sulfur, castor oil packs, activated charcoal and Dmso. These are helpful in binding toxins to ease excretion. A wonderful book by Dr. Amandha Vollmer called "*Healing with DMSO*" is a fantastic resource to learn more.

Diatomaceous earth is the fossilized remains of the shells of freshwater diatoms, which are found in abundance around the world. The micro size shells are mostly composed of silica and are razor sharp to small pathogens such as parasites like fleas, mites and insects. The shells are not large enough to damage human's intestinal tract but they do a great number on bugs. DE works well taken internally and also as a full body mask for things like demodex mites (which we all have, the root cause of acne is mites!!) Also, a super way to prevent fleas on your pets as a monthly dusting on their fur rather than harmful flea medications. Just make sure to keep away from the respiratory tract as it will irritate and can also scratch the eye sclera. When taken internally on a once or twice a week basis it can be part of a fantastic parasite prevention protocol for both you and your beloved furry friends.

That being said a parasite cleanse is and should be part of a seasonal maintenance program. We are naive to think that only animals get parasite and humans do not. Much of the literature mentions that parasite infestations are rare in developed countries- if this is so then why are most parasite medications only available for pets and not for humans? Many vets ask, the moment you enter, "does your pet have flea, tick and heart worm prevention?" But our GPs don't ask us? Old medical and homeopathic books are filled with information on parasites and their contribution to many chronic illnesses and somehow, they have all just disappeared. Why? Every single rife biofeedback scan comes up with multiple parasites and yet current allopathic medicine does not acknowledge this simple fact. We are filled with them and therefore must be prudent to clean and cook our food properly, maintain our pet's health if we have close contact and be sure to do a parasite cleanse at least annually for all members of the family. This is a must!

Parasite cleanses must last for at least two weeks to kill the eggs and adults. But it can be tricky because larvae can actually become immune to whatever herbs or medicines we are using. Much like a bacteria can become resistant to antibiotics. If doing a parasite cleanse for the first time it is wise to change the protocol every two weeks and do the cleanse for 6-8-12 weeks depending on your current health status. Combining herbs like black walnut, clove and wormwood with pumpkin seeds would be a basic

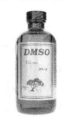 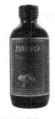 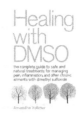
cleanse. Adding MSM sulfur and DMSO and Magnesium would be intermediate. For severe cases dewormers like Ivermectin (see Covid Math plus protocol), Fenbenzadole (see cancer curing abilities), Albendazole and Praziquantanel or Pyrantel Pamoate may be necessary and used with a health practitioner always. Parasites can be very stubborn to eradicate once they have taken up house. Refer to Hulda Clark's book The Cure for All Diseases for more information. Always use muscle testing as a guide for where to go and what methods to use. I find Biofeedback Scans are the fastest confirmation second to biomagnetism. You can find a practitioner on the true rife website.

https://www.curezone.org/cleanse/liver/huldas_recipe.asp
https://us.drclark.com/shop?campaignid=6448079692&adgroupid=79724555249&a-did=437073866371&gclid=Cj0KCQjw0caCBhCIARIsAGAfuMwoMOeCCap0Q2X-qdS4iSMWb8b8ktotowZ562KWC0UiesxENX8_23ZIaAkOGEALw_wcB

The Amazing Liver & Gallbladder Flush by Andreas Moritz
https://www.coseva.com/advanced-trs/

Healing with DMSO by Amandha Vollmer
The Cure for All Diseases by Hulda Clark
https://www.rehabmart.com/product/relax-infrared-situp-sauna-silver-49667.html?gclid=Cj0KCQjw0caCBhCIARIsAGAfuMw9tKbCt8CQFLniCf2a5h-PJmoMFxGTrAWe-hZr5ap0SZfZGhX4XFqQaAmI9EALw_wcB
https://www.ncbi.nlm.nih.gov/pmc/articles/PMC3504417/
https://www.klinik-st-georg.de/en/klinik-st-georg/st-george-hospital/therapies/hyperthermia/

https://www.ncbi.nlm.nih.gov/pmc/articles/PMC2687140/
https://www.pga.com/story/oklahoma-pga-professional-mark-fuller-finds-hope-and-a
https://www.evms.edu/media/evms_public/departments/internal_
medicine/Marik_Critical_Care_COVID-19_Protocol.pdf

11. Colloidal Silver

Aids cure U.S. Patent #5676977 Tetra Silver- Colloidal silver can kill over 650+ disease causing pathogens, including parasites, bacteria, viruses, fungus and yeast. In April 2007, Dr Boyd E. Graves of San Diego visited the Jersey Shore to speak about HIV and AIDS. His thesis presented information about a cure using electrolyzed nano colloidal silver that was injected into critical AIDS patients in Africa as part of a medical study. All but one of the 12 men were permanently cured within one week. Sadly the 12th man passed as he was in the worst condition. The video can be seen here:

https://youtu.be/dsj15rxLTMM

CS is a powerful antimicrobial, effective against a broad spectrum of pathogens it attacks all three of the germs vulnerable targets at once. First the silver ions easily rupture the outer membrane when present in the correct amounts, causing the germs vital internal components to be exposed in the bloodstream to our immune system- our white blood cells. The silver continues to destroy these vital internal components by cutting up vital enzymes inside the pathogen. The silver ions then easily attack the germ's third and most vulnerable target: its DNA. Once the ions combine with the DNA the genes then become paralyzed and the germ cannot reproduce itself.

CS is very simple to make, many rife machines come with silver generators and instructions to follow. It heals pink eye often in a single dose! So much can be said about this amazing molecule. In some countries it has been claimed to heal Marburg viruses such as Ebola. Of course, that information is very difficult to find any longer. Studies showed that wealthy families in the 1700s who ate with silverware had better health and lived longer. Today our flatware is no longer made of silver. It is toxic blends of alloys and leeches' harmful metals into our food and saliva sadly.

A recent study showed that families that dined on silver flatware and dishes had less incidence of disease and a longer life. https://drhealthbenefits.com/lifestyle/healthy/healthy-guide/health-benefits-of-using-silver-utensils

Now very hard to come by but not bad to inherit your great grandmothers old tea set. Etsy still sells some beautiful antiques.

12. MMS/OZONE/Oxygen Therapy

A very critical molecule responsible for optimum health which is probably the most important for disease reduction is good old O2 (see Prana above). Oxygen reduces to water by the mitochondrial electron transport chain and helps supply the metabolic needs of human life. Without proper blood oxygenation anaerobic bacteria are able to thrive due to the suppression of cellular metabolism and turn the area into a hypoxic and toxic soup. It is known that tissue hypoxia is the driving force for cancers heart disease, diabetes, Chronic Fatigue Syndrome, and a host of other health conditions. Ph Balance and Oxygen balance alone are the two greatest predictors of chronic morbidity. Without oxygen, tissues become highly acidic in PH and allow a pooling of toxic molecules that cannot clear out properly. A constant state of inflammation and inflammatory responses by the immune system leads to a break down in structure and function of the cellular systems and eventually to the body as a whole.

Conditions like arthritis, gout, neuropathies, diabetes, anemia, cancer and cardiovascular conditions can all be linked to an imbalance in O2 and pH. Some simple observations demonstrate that people with chronic diseases have ineffective or heavy breathing patterns 24/7. These ineffective breathing patterns cause tissue hypoxia, chronic inflammation, immunosuppression and many other negative effects all caused

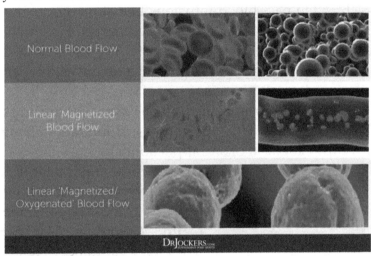

by low body oxygen levels and hypocapnia (reduced CO2 levels). So how do we optimize our uptake of oxygen?

The answers are simple: exercise, increase electricity, proper vitamins and minerals, breathe deeply, and reduce overall intake of things that are highly refined and have an acid pH. These are simple easy and effective ways of preventing chronic illness from happening. But what do we do if we are already sick?? There are many wonderful oxygen therapies available that really do improve health but albeit temporarily. Hyperbaric oxygen therapy has been a crucial tool in helping to fight Lyme disease and its co-infections as well as cancers and lung diseases. Mobile oxygen concentrators like www.inogen.com is a wonderful and affordable way to increase oxygen in those that need constant oxygen supplementation (without a RX) to have a room oxygen reading of 94 or higher on a pulse oximeter (Also a wonderful tool to have in the first aid kit).

As for exercise tools, there is no excuse for fully mobile individuals to not exercise, even if its just a little each day there is ALWAYS time. There are hand bikes, under desk bikes, TRX door systems, home gyms, attachments to turn a regular bike into a stationary bike, aquatic fitness, walking, gardening, even dancing, trampoline rebounding, black mirrors,

Pelotons, Wattbike's, Bowflex systems, lap pools, ergs and the list goes on. Finding something that you enjoy is all that really matters — making it fun and dedicating yourself to your own best health is so important. No one can do it but you!! If you don't use it you lose it. There is freedom in discipline. All it takes is one step in the right direction and the other will follow.

Ozone is another wonderful molecule that has a great many benefits. It can be made in small and practical applications such as an ointment to heal wounds, as a toothpaste for oral health, as kitchen surface disinfectant, and even added to drinking water. Even ozone bulbs can be used on HVAC units to purify air. It also has some very potent medical uses such as ten pass blood infusions like at medical clinics like Infusio or Klinik St Gorg or Sophia Institute. It can also be used in rectal insufflations, oil inhalations, subcutaneous injections and water ozone enemas. The list is long. The only place it cannot be used is in the respiratory tract. It can cause severe asthma attacks and mucosal irritation of the lungs and nasal passages.

For some more amazing info on Ozone see the works of Dr Frank Shallenberger called The Ozone Miracle(lay person basic foundational) and Principle Applications of Ozone Therapy (medical ozone applications).

www.trulyheal.com Marcus Freudmann is a fantastic teacher. I highly recommend his courses. His knowledge is vast. Everything from laser therapies, ozone, rife, saunas and more. He has great intro courses for the functional medicine practitioner and more.

https://youtu.be/-UoLB6SprdM
https://youtu.be/oHQBSnszTlA
www.ozonegenerator.com
www.trulyheal.com

MMS is a step above ozone therapy. It is highly controversial to most that have not researched its amazing benefits. Mainstream media has painted it in a bad light. Yes, it could be categorized as a bleach like chemical and used in similar applications. However, when one studies the chemistry of MMS they will quickly understand that it is a naturally occurring substance in the human body. It can kill pathogens in a very short time. It can kill cancer cells by introducing an oxygen rich environment. It can kill fungus and bacteria as well as parasites and their eggs. It can kill viruses also. The key is knowing how to use it "Properly ". Proper dosage is key.

There are a few methods available but again these methods are being suppressed by corporate government bodies. It is somewhat precautionary for good reason. When mixing chemicals, it should really require someone who fully understands chemistry and how to properly handle these substances. It requires proper glass equipment, ventilation and more. The idea behind MMS is activating two substances that off gas oxygen into the body and thus killing anything that thrives anaerobically. This substance must be micro dosed.

When used effectively it can cure ALL diseases. Yes all.

For more information research Jim Humbles protocol 1000 MMS. His "church" has recently been quashed and his books are now difficult to obtain. There is also an amazing chemist named Andreas Kalcker who has revived and improved Humbles methods. His $30 course online should be a first step into exploring MMS and how to use it.

Recently Dr. Robert O Young has come forth with an even better way to use Sodium Hypochlorite as a 5 percent solution in distilled water without activation (see Dr Gregorio Placeres autism work. MMS sin activar). This I believe is the most sound chemical method of application, allowing the stomach acid to activate the MMS thus off gassing the oxygen into the cells of the body to cure acidic and toxic imbalances.

The protocols of these methods are all similar with slight differences. Bottom line. Take caution and use as directed

Due to censorship it would also be prudent to archive the information you have. Anything that can actually truly cure an illness is a threat to the pharmaceutical business and will be eliminated. So save hard copies or storage drives with this info. It disappears daily.

www.andreaskalcker.com
https://youtu.be/Dt1KexkADgY
https://jimhumble.co
http://www.altcancer.com
http://www.mmsmineralshop.com
https://www.fda.gov/inspections-compliance-enforcement-and-criminal-investigations/warning-letters/genesis-2-church-606459-04082020
Robert O Young Ph *Miracle books*

13. Mineral Depletion

Our agricultural practices have been intended to create "fast food". Food that grows fast in any conditions and produces huge yields with little nutrients. A bell pepper from 1930 compared to 2020 is ten times weaker in all its minerals. Soils are lacking in iodine, selenium, boron, magnesium and more. Most people today are deficient in magnesium which is critical for 90 chemically energetic processes in our body. It burns bright white and when it does it creates energy potentials in our cells. Without magnesium we develop Early signs of deficiency including loss of appetite, nausea, vomiting, fatigue, hypertension and weakness. As magnesium deficiency worsens, numbness, tingling, muscle contractions and cramps, seizures, personality changes, abnormal heart rhythms, and coronary spasms can occur. Magnesium relaxes smooth muscle tissue and is necessary for relaxation in our bodies. A simple pure Epsom salt bath mixed with sea salt for 20 minutes up to the neck in hot water once a week will be the best way to get such a critical mineral into the body. (orally it can cause diarrhea so transdermal is best).

Another important mineral is boron. It has been shown in medical studies to decrease urinary output of calcium in women up to 40 percent in one dose in osteoporosis patients. See Andreas Kalckers book *Salud Prohibidad* for more dosing information.

14. Iodine

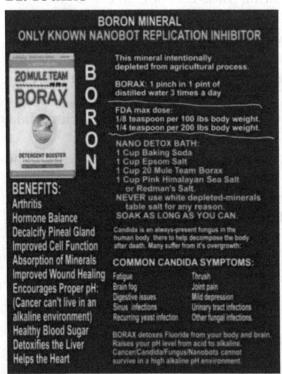

Another critical mineral. It is responsible for the formation of ALL of our hormones and directly related to the thyroid and its imbalances. Halides like fluoride, chlorine and bromine also fit in iodine receptors and are stronger than iodine. They basically override the absorption of iodine and prevent hormones from being made efficiently. If you have thyroid or hormone issues. Remove toxic table salt from your diet immediately and read the book "Iodine Crisis" by Lynne Farrow. I do not recommend Iodoral however I do love her info and fully support nascent iodine supplements and or lugols iodine. To see if you are deficient do a simple skin test. Firstly, to see if you are allergic (it is rare but serious). If the patch is absorbed within 24 hours you have a need for more iodine in your body. Nascent iodine is best for beginners as a raindrop therapy and is safe for vulnerable populations.

Lugols is stronger and would be a step up after a year of using nascent iodine. One drop in water on an empty stomach, early morning rising. Taken away from vitamin C as iodine will lose its antimicrobial abilities. Usually a two-hour window is sufficient.

IOSAT tablets are also not a bad idea to have in an emergency kit. Especially anyone who works in nuclear energy careers.

The same company that makes magnesium also sells the iodine. Borax can be purchased online or at your local supermarket.

15. Iron

See Dr. Sebi and his work on Irish Sea Moss. It is an amazing superfood high in the best iron and bromine- to be taken away from iodine and with vitamin C to enhance its effects.

16. Vitamin C

We are the only mammal on the planet that does not make our own. Gorillas, when injured can make up to 22,000 mg per day. Most animals make more when injured and do not need to get any from outside sources. Vitamin C is necessary for healthy collagen formation and immune support as well as effective oxygenation of red blood cells. It facilitates all healthy tissue repair. Without it our skin does not heal properly. The best type of Vitamin C is liposomal. It mimicks IV administration and in some studies performs better than IV methods. Make sure to use a brand that does not have GMO or soy. Liponaturals sunflower brand is wonderful https://liponaturals.com

Other kinds of vitamin C are good also. A buffered kind is best as it keeps the body alkaline such as Calcium Ascorbate or sodium ascorbate by https://biomedicine.com/ProductDetail/35011070_The-Right-C--100-Grams

Studies show high amounts of vitamin C prior to surgery of any kind prevents excessive bleeding and promotes faster healing up to 50 percent.

https://www.ancient-minerals.com

https://shop.enviromedica.com/nascent-iodine-product-details

17. Fulvic Acid

Shilajit or Mumyio is a tar like substance harvested at the top of mountains that contains trace minerals and fulvic acid.

Shilajit contains more than 84 minerals, so it offers numerous health benefits. It can function as an antioxidant to improve your body's immunity and memory, an anti-inflammatory, an energy booster, and a diuretic to remove excess fluid from your body. It tastes like tar and salted black licorice and comes in many forms. It is truly amazing the benefits of this ancient superfood if you feel you are looking to up your minerals or balance your electrolytes.

Cymbiotika Shilajit - Black Gold Recurring, Cancel Anytime (USD 58.00)$58.00cymbiotika.com

18. Dry Brushing

Ancients knew the benefits of brushing the body for health. The lymphatics have no valves therefore they do not push lymph through the body without movement of facilitating muscles. If you don't move the immune system doesn't flow. See the video " the Fuzz" for more on stagnation and what happens when we do not do bodywork. Dry Brushing is done from the extremities inward and towards the heart. Once a week it can be super invigorating and beneficial to places that we don't give much attention.

Heavy Metal Detox Foods

This is an excerpt from my book, "Geoengineering aka Chemtrails". Due to ever constant aerosol spraying of toxins from the air, we are almost daily ingesting nanoparticulate heavy metals. These superfoods will help lift and detox out of your system.

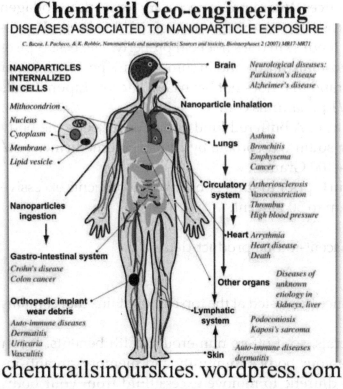

Chemtrail Geo-engineering
DISEASES ASSOCIATED TO NANOPARTICLE EXPOSURE

C. Buzea, I. Pacheco, & K. Robbie, Nanomaterials and nanoparticles: Sources and toxicity, Biointerphases 2 (2007) MR17-MR71

NANOPARTICLES INTERNALIZED IN CELLS

Mithocondrion
Nucleus
Cytoplasm
Membrane
Lipid vesicle

Nanoparticles ingestion

Gastro-intestinal system
Crohn's disease
Colon cancer

Orthopedic implant wear debris
Auto-immune diseases
Dermatitis
Urticaria
Vasculitis

Brain — Neurological diseases: Parkinson's disease, Alzheimer's disease

Nanoparticle inhalation

Lungs — Asthma, Bronchitis, Emphysema, Cancer

Circulatory system — Artheriosclerosis, Vasoconstriction, Thrombus, High blood pressure

Heart — Arrythmia, Heart disease, Death

Other organs — Diseases of unknown etiology in kidneys, liver

Lymphatic system — Podoconiosis, Kaposi's sarcoma

Skin — Auto-immune diseases, dermatitis

chemtrailsinourskies.wordpress.com

1. **Spirulina** is an edible blue-green algae. It is known for its distinctive green color and strong odor and delivers a strong dose of protein, all eight of the essential amino acids, iron, folic acid, B vitamins, selenium and manganese, resulting in strong **therapeutic benefits**. Spirulina can be effective in removing heavy metals from the nervous system and the liver.

2. **Chlorella** is a solid green-colored form of algae. Although it is a little harder to digest than spirulina, **chlorella is known to be effective in removing heavy metals** for just this reason. Chlorella's cell walls are very tough and often cannot be fully digested, and it is these cell walls that bind to toxins in your body in order to eliminate them.

3. **Atlantic dulse** is edible seaweed that binds to metals such as aluminum (which is extremely prevalent in the food industry), mercury, lead, copper and nickel. This seaweed works in the digestive tract all the way through the colon to seek out and bind with toxic heavy metals, without releasing them back into the body.

4. **Barley grass juice powder** is not a very common food, but it does help address heavy metals toxicity in the various parts of the digestive system and the reproductive organs. If **coupled with spirulina, barley grass juice powder can be even more effective**.

5. **Edible wild plants dandelion and milk thistle** both cleanse the blood vessels and improve the functionality of the liver, which is an important organ when it comes to eliminating impurities from the body.

6. **Ginger** is one of the healthiest plants on Earth. In addition to improving digestion and reducing inflammation in the body, ginger root supports kidney function. The kidneys play an important role in the body's elimination process and are often one of the first targets of heavy metals toxicity, so they need ginger's extra power boost.

7. **Artichokes**: Artichokes help the liver function at its best, which in turn will help your body purge itself of toxins and other things it doesn't need to survive. It ups the liver's production of bile, and since bile helps break down foods which helps your body use the nutrients inside them, an increase in bile production is typically a good thing.

8. **Organic Apples**: Apples are full of wonderful nutrients. You get fiber, vitamins, minerals and many beneficial phytochemicals such as D-Glucarate, flavonoids and terpenoids. All of these substances are used in the detox process. One flavonoid, Phlorizidin (phlorizin), is thought to help stimulate bile production which helps with detox as the liver gets rid of some toxins through the bile. Apples are also a good source of the soluble fiber pectin, which can help detox metals and food additives from your body. It's best to eat only organic apples as the non-organic varieties are among the top 12 foods that have been found to contain the most pesticide residues. Organically produced apples also have a 15 percent higher antioxidant capacity than conventionally produced apples.

9. **Almonds:** Almonds are the best nut source of Vitamin E. In fact, just one ounce contains 7.3 mg of "alpha-tocopheral" vitamin E, the form of the vitamin the body prefers. They're also high in fiber, calcium, magnesium, and useable protein that helps stabilize blood sugar and remove impurities from the bowels.

10. **Asparagus**: Not only does asparagus help to detoxify the body, it can help you wage the anti-aging battle, protect you from getting cancer, help your heart to stay healthy, and is a general anti-inflammatory food. It's also known to help with liver drainage, which might sound like a bad thing, but since the liver is responsible for filtering out the toxic materials in the food and drinks we consume, anything that backs up its drainage is not doing you any favors. Asparagus also helps reduce risk of death from breast cancer and increase the odds of survival.

11. **Avocados**: This wonder fruit is packed with antioxidants, lowers cholesterol and dilates the blood vessels while blocking artery-destroying toxicity. Avocados contain a nutrient called glutathione, which blocks at least 30 different carcinogens while helping the liver detoxify synthetic chemicals. Researchers at the University of Michigan found that elderly people who had high levels of glutathione were healthier and less likely to suffer from arthritis. Consuming avocados is associated with better diet quality and nutrient intake level, lower intake of added sugars, lower body weight, BMI and waist circumferences, higher "good cholesterol" levels and lower metabolic syndrome risk.

12. **Basil**: Basil has anti-bacterial properties, and it's full of antioxidants to protect the liver. The active ingredients are terpenoids. It is also wonderful for digestion and detoxification, too. It supports the functioning of the kidneys and also acts as a diuretic to help the body expel unwanted toxins. Basil has been known to have anti-ulcer qualities as well as antimicrobial effects that guard against bacteria, yeast, fungi and mold. Basil seed can also help with constipation. The anitcancer properties of basil may also relate to its ability to influence viral infections.

13. **Beets**: A single serving of beets can do more for your health than most foods in the produce isle. Not only can they boost your energy and lower your blood pressure, but eating beets in the long-term can help you fight cancer, reduce arthritic pain, boost your brain as well as help you lose weight. Beets contain a unique mixture of natural plant chemicals (phytochemicals) and minerals that make them superb fighters of infection, blood purifiers, and liver cleansers. They also help boost the body's cellular intake of oxygen, making beets excellent overall body cleansers. When you're detoxing, beets will help by making sure that the toxins you're getting out actually make it out of your body. Many detox cleanses go wrong when toxins are reintroduced to the body because they don't make it all the way out.

14. Blueberries: Blueberries contain natural aspirin that helps lessen the tissue-damaging effects of chronic inflammation, while lessening pain. Just 300 grams of blueberries protects against DNA damage. Blueberries also act as antibiotics by blocking bacteria in the urinary tract, thereby helping to prevent infections. They have antiviral properties and are loaded with super-detoxifying phytonutrients called proanthocyanidins.

15. Brazil Nuts: These tasty treats are packed with selenium, which is key to flushing mercury out of your body. The body uses selenium to make 'selenoproteins', which work like antioxidants preventing damage to cells and there is growing body of evidence to show it has a key role in our health. The consumption of brazil nuts has been found to be inversely associated with risk of pancreatic cancer, independent of other potential risk factors for pancreatic cancer.

16. Broccoli: Broccoli specifically works with the enzymes in your liver to turn toxins into something your body can eliminate easily. If you're stuck for ways on how to make broccoli taste better try dehydrating or consider eating it raw. But don't microwave it as this destroys both the nutritional and detox potential. Broccoli contains a very powerful anti-cancer, anti-diabetic and anti-microbial called sulforaphame which helps prevent cancer, diabetes, osteoporosis and allergies.

17. Broccoli Sprouts: Broccoli sprouts can actually provide more benefit than regular broccoli as they contain 20 times more sulforophane. They contain important phytochemicals that are released when they're chopped, chewed, fermented, or digested. The substances are released then break down into sulforophanes, indole-3-carbinol and D-glucarate, which all have a specific effect on detoxification. Add these to your salads and get creative with them in your meals. Researchers have found that an oral preparation made from broccoli sprouts trigger an increase in inflammation-fighting enzymes in the upper airways.

18. Cabbage: In addition to cleansing your liver, cabbage will also aid in helping you go to the bathroom, which in turn helps you expel the toxins, getting them out of your system so you can start fresh. It contains sulfur, which is essential when it comes to breaking down chemicals and removing them from your body. Along with other cold crops, cabbage is a source of indole-3-carbinol, a chemical that boosts DNA repair in cells and appears to block the growth of cancer cells.

19. Cilantro: Cilantro, also known as coriander, Chinese parsley or dhania, contains an abundance of anitoxidants. Cilantro helps mobilize mercury and other metals out of the tissue so it can attach to it other compounds and allow it to be excreted from the body. It also contains an antibacterial compound called dodecenal, which laboratory tests showed is twice as effective as the commonly used antibiotic drug gentamicin at killing Salmonella.

20. Cinnamon: The oils from cinnamon contain active components called cinnamalde-hyde, cinnamyl acetate, and cinnamyl alcohol. Cinnamaldehyde has been well-researched for its effects on blood platelets helps prevent unwanted clumping of blood cells. Cinnamon's essential oils also qualify it as an "anti-microbial" food, and cinnamon has been studied for its ability to help stop the growth of bacteria as well as fungi, including the commonly problematic yeast Candida. Cinnamon's antimicrobial properties are so effective that recent research demonstrates this spice can be used as an alternative to traditional food preservatives. It has one of the highest antioxidant values of all foods and its use in medicine treats everything from nausea to menstruation and energy to diabetes.

21. Cranberries: While they are more popular as fruits that help prevent urinary tract infections, cranberries are antibacterial and are known to remove many different toxins from your body. Cranberries feature a rich profile of anti-inflammatory nutrients, provide immune and cardiovascular support, as well as promote digestive health. Consuming cranberry products has been associated with the prevention of urinary tract infections (UTIs) for over 100 years.

22. Fennel: The fennel bulb is high in fiber may also be useful in preventing colon cancer. In addition to its fiber, fennel is a very good source of folate, a B vitamin that is necessary for the conversion of a dangerous molecule called homocysteine into other, benign mole-cules. The vitamin C found in fennel bulb is directly antimicrobial and is also needed for the proper function of the immune system.

23. Flaxseeds: When detoxifying your body, it's essential to ensure toxins are elimi-nated properly. Ground flaxseeds provide a wonderful source of fiber that helps to bind and flush toxins from the intestinal tract. They're also a great source of health promoting omega 3 oils. Try consuming two tablespoons of ground flaxseeds in lemon water every morning. University of Copenhagen researchers report that flax fiber suppresses appe-tite and helps support weight loss. Men should be cautious when consuming flax as the lignans are similar to the female hormone estrogen as can cause problems for some men.

24. **Garlic:** Many detox diets list garlic as a crucial piece of the puzzle. The reason is that garlic boosts the immune system as well as helping out the liver. One good thing about garlic is that you can up your intake without having to worry if your body is going to get used to it or build up a resistance. Sulfur is found in high quantities in garlic — which makes it a good detox food and its antibiotic properties heal your body. Garlic is proven to be 100 times more effective than antibiotics and working in a fraction of the time.

25. **Goji Berries**: Replace raisins with nutrient-dense Goji berries to boost your vitamin C and beta-carotene intake. Gram for gram, goji berries pack more vitamin C than oranges

and more beta-carotene than carrots. Vitamin C can help remove waste from your body, while beta-carotene improves liver performance.

26. **Grapefruit**: Grapefruits can prevent weight gain, treat diabetes, lower cholesterol, fight cancer, heal stomach ulcers, reduce gum disease and even keep stroke and metabolic syndrome at bay. Grapefruits can treat disease as well as pharmaceuticals without the side effects. The rich pink and red colors of grapefruit are due to lycopene, a carotenoid phytonutrient. Among the common dietary carotenoids, lycopene has the highest capacity to help fight oxygen free radicals, which are compounds that can damage cells. The big takeaway on grapefruit is that it gets your liver fired up and ready for action, while infusing the rest of your organs with nutrient-laden fruit juice.

27. **Green Tea**: Green tea is often thought of as a great addition to any detox program because of its high antioxidant value. It is the least processed tea and thus provides the most antioxidant polyphenols, notably a catechin called epigallocatechin-3-gallate (EGCG), which is believed to be responsible for most of the health benefits linked to green tea. According to 17 clinical trials, green tea is linked with significantly lower blood sugar.

28. **Hemp**: Hemp might just be one of nature's most perfect foods since it is full of anti-oxidants like Vitamins E and C, as well as chlorophyll which is wonderful for cleansing the body from toxins of all kinds, including heavy metals. The soluble and insoluble fiber in hemp can also keep the digestive tract clean and therefore, reduce the toxic burden on other internal organs. Hemp could free us from oil, prevent deforestation, cure cancer and its environmentally beneficial.

29. **Kale**: Kale is now recognized as providing comprehensive support for the body's detoxification system. New research has shown that the ITCs made from kale's gluco-sinolates can help regulate detox at a genetic level. This vegetable is so good for you that it is often recommended to patients that are following a doctor recommended diet when fighting kidney disease. It's packed with so many antioxidants and has anti-inflammatory properties as well, not to mention all of the vitamins and minerals it contains. Leafy greens are likely the number one food you can eat to regularly improve your health. They're filled with fiber along with crucial vitamins, minerals, and plant-based phytochemicals that may help protect you from almost every disease known.

26. **Lemongrass**: This is an herb that is used in Thailand and other parts of the world as a natural way to cleanse several organs at once. It not only helps the liver but also the kidneys, the bladder, and the entire digestive tract. Benefits of using it in your cooking, or drinking it as a tea include a better complexion, better circulation, and better digestion. It is most often used as a tea in the world of detoxing, and there are several recipes you can try until you find one that suits your tastes best.

30. **Lemons**: This wonderful fruit stimulates the release of enzymes and helps convert toxins into a water-soluble form that can be easily excreted from the body. In addition,

they contain high amounts of vitamin C, a vitamin needed by the body to make gluta-thione. Glutathione helps ensure that phase 2 liver detoxification keeps pace with phase 1, thereby reducing the likelihood of negative effects from environmental chemicals. Drinking lemon water, which is alkaline-forming, first thing in the morning will help to balance out the acidity of foods we've consumed. They also have an incredible effect in detoxing the liver. Fresh lemon juice contains more than 20 anti-cancer compounds and helps balance the body's pH levels.

31. **Olive Oil**: Some liver cleanses out there call for olive oil mixed with fruit juice in order to trigger your liver to expunge its gallstones. But aside from that olive oil should be your go-to oil when you're trying to detox the body. That's because it has a lot of healthy properties and makes for a better choice of fat than most of your other options. Just be sure not to cook with it at high heat. Use it as a salad dress to help things like dark leafy greens go down. Your best choice is always ice-pressed olive oil, but if you can find a very high quality cold-pressed olive oil, although not as nutritious, it will suffice provided the quality is high and not adulterated.

32. **Onions**: This ubiquitous kitchen staple is as healthy as it is tasty. It's brimming with sulfur-containing amino acids, which efficiently detox the liver. Raw onions deliver the most health benefits. Even a small amount of "overpeeling" can result in unwanted loss of flavonoids. For example, a red onion can lose about 20% of its quercetin and almost 75% of its anthocyanins if it is "overpeeled". Onions will soak up arsenic, cadmium, lead, mercury and tin in food containers. The total polyphenol content of onion is not only higher than its fellow allium vegetables, garlic and leeks, but also higher than tomatoes, carrots, and red bell pepper. Onions have been shown to inhibit the activity of macrophages, specialized white blood cells that play a key role in our body's immune defense system, and one of their defense activities involves the triggering of large-scale inflammatory responses.

33. **Parsley**: Those pretty green leaves don't just make your plate look great. Parsley boasts plenty of beta-carotene and vitamins A, C and K to protect your kidneys and bladder. Diuretic herbs such as parsley prevent problems such as kidney stones and bladder infec-tions and keep our body's plumbing running smoothly by causing it to produce more urine. They also relieve bloating during menstruation. The flavonoids in parsley–especially luteolin–have been shown to function as antioxidants that combine with highly reactive oxygen-containing molecules (called oxygen radicals) and help prevent oxygen-based damage to cells. In addition, extracts from parsley have been used in animal studies to help increase the antioxidant capacity of the blood.

34. **Pineapples**: This tropical delight contains bromelain, a digestive enzyme that helps cleanse your colon and improve digestion. Excessive inflammation, excessive coagulation of the blood, and certain types of tumor growth may all be reduced by bromelain. Two

molecules isolated from an extract of crushed pineapple stems have even shown promise in fighting cancer growth.

35. **Seaweed**: Seaweed may be the most underrated vegetable in the Western world. Studies at McGill University in Montreal showed that seaweeds bind to radioactive waste in the body so it can be removed. Radioactive waste can find its way into the body through some medical tests or through food that has been grown where water or soil is contaminated. Seaweed also binds to heavy metals to help eliminate them from the body. In addition, it is a powerhouse of minerals and trace minerals. Seaweed extracts can help you lose weight, mostly body fat.

36. **Sesame Seeds**: Sesame seeds' phytosterols have beneficial effects which are so dramatic that they have been extracted from many foods and added to processed foods, such as "butter"-replacement spreads, which are then touted as cholesterol-lowering "foods." But why settle for an imitation "butter" when Mother Nature's nuts and seeds are a naturally rich source of phytosterols–and cardio-protective fiber, minerals and healthy fats as well? Sesame seeds contain minerals important in a number of anti-inflammatory and antioxidant enzyme systems.

37. **Turmeric**: Curcumin is the active ingredient in the spice turmeric, which gives it its yellow color. The rate at which your detox pathways function depends on your genes, your age, lifestyle and a good supply of nutrients involved in the detox process. Curcumin is used a lot in Ayurvedic Medicine to treat liver and digestive disorders. Turmeric has specifically been studied in relation to the positive effect that it has on the liver. As a high antioxidant spice, turmeric protects the body and prevents disease and prevents disease more effectively than drug based treatments and without side effects.

38. **Watercress**: Give your liver a big boost with cleansing action of watercress. If you're into making smoothies for your detoxing this is a great one to blend up and drink down. This helps to release enzymes in the liver that clean it out and help rid it of toxic buildup. Eating watercress each day helps prevent breast cancer.

39. **Wheatgras**s: Wheatgrass restores alkalinity to the blood. The juice's abundance of alkaline minerals helps reduce over-acidity in the blood and thus also Is a powerful detoxifier, and liver protector. It increases red blood-cell count and lowers blood pressure. It also cleanses the organs and gastrointestinal tract of debris. Wheatgrass stimulates the metabolism and the body's enzyme systems by enriching the blood. It also aids in reducing blood pressure by dilating the blood pathways throughout the body. Pound for pound, wheatgrass is more than twenty times denser nutrients than other choice vegetables. Nutritionally, wheatgrass is a complete food that contains 98 of the 102 earth elements. For a full body detox to reduce acidity in the body with wheat grass, organic juices, bentonite clay, celery, cilantro, and fruits and vegetables. Ginko biloba, cayenne pepper, and turmeric help. Vitamin D is similar to 'sun in a bottle', an immune booster,

and vitamin of the future. Humans should consume baking soda and lemon juice in their body often to alkalize themselves.

Apple Cider Vinegar is highly beneficial. Hypothyroidism occurs from iodine-deficiency and can be combated and cured with Iodine. *IODINE* is found in organic homegrown garcinia cambogia, neem, spirulina, algae, kelp, seaweed, and chlorella. Coconut oil can be rubbed on the thyroid and pineal gland frequently.

Diatomaceous Clay removes heavy metal toxins as well including radiation. You can eat it and bathing in it is very helpful as well. These foods will assist in boosting your metabolism, optimizing digestion, while allowing you to lose weight and fortify your immune system.

Throw out all toxic cleaners under your kitchen sink and bathrooms. You can make your own home health cleaners with apple cider vinegar, baking soda, borax, organic lemon juice and essential oils. See below section for formulas of different ways to make your own home cleaners. **Make your own home cleaners:**

http://tiphero.com/homemade-cleaning-products-for-all-your-cleaning-needs/

In addition, one should always protect themselves, and loved ones, by wearing hats to cover their heads whenever aerosol spraying is occurring. This will also help with protecting against the cancer causing UVB rays bombarding Earth's inhabitants as well. Staying indoors on heavy aerosol spraying days is another good idea whenever possible. To be very clear, it is our children, with their still-developing immune systems who are most at risk due to GE practices, so getting them to eat healthy, biodynamic or organic local food is imperative.

Cannabis Cures Cancer
...and Nearly Everything Else

THC (marijuana) helps cure cancer says Harvard Study

The term medical marijuana took on dramatic new meaning in February 2000 when researchers in Madrid announced they had destroyed incurable brain cancer tumors in rats by injecting them with THC, the active ingredient in cannabis.

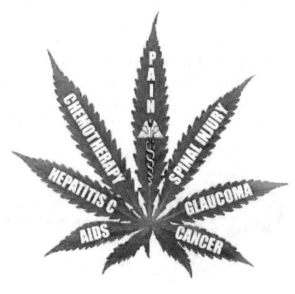

The Madrid study marks only the second time that THC has been administered to tumor-bearing animals; the first was a Virginia investigation 26 years ago. In both studies, the THC shrank or destroyed tumors in a majority of the test subjects.

Most Americans don't know anything about the Madrid discovery. Virtually no U.S. newspapers carried the story, which ran only once on the AP and UPI news wires, on Feb. 29.

The ominous part is that this isn't the first time scientists have discovered that THC shrinks tumors. In 1974 researchers at the Medical College of Virginia, who had been funded by the National Institute of Health to find evidence that marijuana damages the immune system, found instead that THC slowed the growth of three kinds of cancer in mice — lung and breast cancer, and a virus-induced leukemia.

The DEA quickly shut down the Virginia study and all further cannabis/tumor research, according to Jack Herer, who reports on the events in his book, "The Emperor Wears No Clothes". In 1976 President Gerald Ford put an end to all public cannabis research and granted exclusive research rights to major pharmaceutical companies, who set out — unsuccessfully — to develop synthetic forms of THC that would deliver all the medical benefits without the "high."

The Madrid researchers reported in the March issue of "Nature Medicine" that they injected the brains of 45 rats with cancer cells, producing tumors whose presence they confirmed through magnetic resonance imaging (MRI). On the 12th day they injected 15 of the rats with THC and 15 with Win-55,212-2 a synthetic compound similar to THC.

"All the rats left untreated uniformly died 12-18 days after glioma (brain cancer) cell inoculation ... Cannabinoid (THC)-treated rats survived significantly longer than control rats. THC administration was ineffective in three rats, which died by days 16-18. Nine of the THC-treated rats surpassed the time of death of untreated rats, and survived up to 19-35 days. Moreover, the tumor was completely eradicated in three of the treated rats." The rats treated with Win-55,212-2 showed similar results.

The Spanish researchers, led by Dr. Manuel Guzman of Complutense University, also irrigated healthy rats' brains with large doses of THC for seven days, to test for harmful biochemical or neurological effects. They found none.

"Careful MRI analysis of all those tumor-free rats showed no sign of damage related to necrosis, edema, infection or trauma ... We also examined other potential side effects of cannabinoid administration. In both tumor-free and tumor-bearing rats, cannabinoid administration induced no substantial change in behavioral parameters such as motor

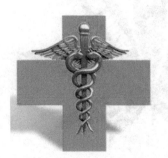

coordination or physical activity. Food and water intake as well as body weight gain were unaffected during and after cannabinoid delivery. Likewise, the general hematological profiles of cannabinoid-treated rats were normal.

Thus, neither biochemical parameters nor markers of tissue damage changed substantially during the 7-day delivery period or for at least 2 months after cannabinoid treatment ended."

Guzman's investigation is the only time since the 1974 Virginia study that THC has been administered to live tumor-bearing animals. (The Spanish researchers cite a 1998 study in which cannabinoids inhibited breast cancer cell proliferation, but that was a "petri dish" experiment that didn't involve live subjects.)

In an email interview for this story, the Madrid researcher said he had heard of the Virginia study, but had never been able to locate literature on it. Hence, the Nature Medicine article characterizes the new study as the first on tumor-laden animals and doesn't cite the 1974 Virginia investigation.

"I am aware of the existence of that research. In fact I have attempted many times to obtain the journal article on the original investigation by these people, but it has proven impossible." Guzman said:

In 1983 the Reagan/Bush Administration tried to persuade American universities and researchers to destroy all 1966-76 cannabis research work, including compendiums in libraries, reports Jack Herer, who states, "We know that large amounts of information have since disappeared."

Guzman provided the title of the work — "Antineoplastic activity of cannabinoids," an article in a 1975 Journal of the National Cancer Institute — and this writer obtained a copy at the UC medical school library in Davis and faxed it to Madrid.

The summary of the Virginia study begins, "Lewis lung adenocarcinoma growth was retarded by the oral administration of tetrahydrocannabinol (THC) and cannabinol (CBN)" — two types of cannabinoids, a family of active components in marijuana. "Mice treated for 20 consecutive days with THC and CBN had reduced primary tumor size."

The 1975 journal article doesn't mention breast cancer tumors,

which featured in the only newspaper story ever to appear about the 1974 study — in the Local section of the Washington Post on August 18, 1974. Under the headline, "Cancer Curb Is Studied," it read in part:

"The active chemical agent in marijuana curbs the growth of three kinds of cancer in mice and may also suppress the immunity reaction that causes rejection of organ transplants, a Medical College of Virginia team has discovered."

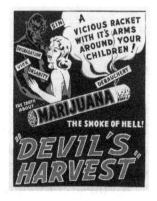

The researchers "found that THC slowed the growth of lung cancers, breast cancers and a virus-induced leukemia in laboratory mice and prolonged their lives by as much as 36 percent."

Guzman, writing from Madrid, was eloquent in his response after this writer faxed him the clipping from the Washington Post of a quarter century ago. In translation, he wrote:

"It is extremely interesting to me, the hope that the project seemed to awaken at that moment, and the sad evolution (lastimosa evolucion) of events during the years following the discovery, until now we once again draw back the veil over the anti-tumoral power of THC, twenty-five years later. Unfortunately, the world bumps along between such moments of hope and long periods of intellectual castration."

News coverage of the Madrid discovery has been virtually nonexistent in this country. The news broke quietly on Feb. 29, [2000] with a story that ran once on the UPI wire about the Nature Medicine article. This writer stumbled on it through a link that appeared briefly on the Drudge Report web page.

The New York Times, Washington Post and Los Angeles Times all ignored the story, even though its newsworthiness is indisputable: a benign substance occurring in nature destroys deadly brain tumors.

"Why is marijuana against the law? It grows naturally upon our planet. Doesn't the idea of making nature against the law seem to you a bit . . . unnatural?" — Bill Hicks

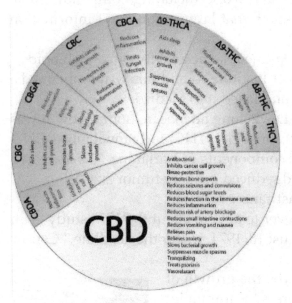

CBG-A, or Cannabigerolic Acid is the primordial phyto-cannabinoid. It is the compound in cannabis from which all the plant's other naturally occurring cannabinoids are formed : without CBGA, the cannabis plant cannot produce its most useful compounds.

Despite this obvious importance, it still remains one of the most under-studied cannabinoids, with the majority of current research focusing on the healing properties of THC, CBD and CBN.

Here we aim to elucidate some of the important features of this 'building block' cannabinoid to demonstrate why exactly it deserves more attention in the medical cannabis community.

CBGA & Beyond

As mentioned in the introduction, all cannabinoids begin life as CBGA. There is then a biosynthesis within the plant's cells involving certain enzymes that dictate whether that compound goes on to become Cannabidiolic Acid (CBDA), Tetrahydrocannabinolic Acid (THCA) or less commonly, remain as Cannabigerolic Acid (CBGA) or become Cannabichromene Acid (CBCA).

All these compounds are still in their raw, acidic form, hence the 'A' which denotes the molecule having an acid component. The molecule in this raw state carries a carbon ring in its outer layer that dictates its appearance as an acid.

The traditional course of action to prepare cannabinoids for consumption is to heat and thus 'decarboxylate' (remove the outer carbon ring from the molecule by subjecting it to heat) the molecules. This process converts THCA into THC, CBDA into CBD and CBCA into CBC.

The reason this process is usually performed is that cannabinoids in raw, acidic forms do not create the psychoactive effects in the human body that heated or 'decarboxylated' cannabinoids do.

However, this can benefit medical patients: as there is no physical or psychological effect when consumed, much greater quantities can be consumed in a single dose.

Raw cannabinoid therapy is in its infancy but shows potential to be an effective way of getting large quantities of cannabinoids into the body without the psychoactive effects that can be unpleasant for some. More details and particulars are discussed in this interview with a pioneer of raw cannabis medicine, Dr. William Courtney.

Aside from the pathways CBGA can take in its biosynthesis journey to become CBDA,THCA or CBCA, there are further permutations caused by environmental factors that create other, different cannabinoids.

First, CBGA can also undergo the same decarboxylation or heating to become CBG.

Though it is usually only found in negligible quantities when testing harvested cannabis flowers - possibly due to much of CBGA being converted into other cannabinoids by the plant's own mechanisms - its properties are not to be underestimated. CBG has been shown to help reduce inflammation, intraocular pressure, anxiety and depression; along with demonstrating synergistic effects alongside other cannabinoids to improve overall efficacy.

These findings alone should be enough to make the case for further study of its potential medical value, yet it continues to receive less attention than its more famous cousins, THC, CBD and CBN.

CBGA is starting to pique the interest of more cannabis breeders with each passing month : much like the Stanley Brothers became seen as pioneers of CBD-rich cultivars, companies like TGA Seeds (started by renowned breeder 'Subcool') are experimenting with trying to develop CBG-rich cultivars. This has been made possible by selecting cannabis plants that already demonstrated greater-than-average CBGA production and pollinating them with certain industrial hemp plants.

The industrial hemp plants selected for these breeding experiments naturally demonstrate a higher CBGA profile, resulting in offspring that retain higher CBGA levels in the cannabis flower.

So as the precursor to all other cannabinoids, a molecule shown to have positive synergy with said cannabinoids and a valuable compound in its own right; CBGA has an excellent case to be the next major phyto-cannabinoid to receive attention from researchers.

Though there is research around CBGA, it currently focuses on trying to decipher what processes are taking place within the trichomes of the cannabis plant - to be able to better explain how CBGA becomes THCA, CBDA and others - rather than on its medicinal potential.

With more breeders selecting cultivars for increased CBGA production, it's promising percentages in industrial hemp plants, and information becoming more readily available on the potential of this cannabinoid, we should begin to see more data supporting CBGA's possible role as a primary cannabinoid in treating a variety of diseases.

As detailed in Part I of this article, the health benefits of cannabis are now well established. It is a cheap, natural alternative effective for a broad range of conditions, and the non-psychoactive form known as hemp has thousands of industrial uses. At one time, cannabis was one of the world's most important crops. There have been no recorded deaths from cannabis overdose in the US, compared to about 30,000 deaths annually from alcohol abuse (not counting auto accidents), and 100,000 deaths annually from prescription drugs taken as directed. Yet cannabis remains a Schedule I controlled substance ("a deadly dangerous drug with no medical use and high potential for abuse"), illegal to be sold or grown in the US.

Powerful corporate interests no doubt had a hand in keeping cannabis off the market. The question now is why they have suddenly gotten on the bandwagon for its legalization. According to an April 2014 article in The Washington Times, the big money behind the recent push for legalization has come, not from a grassroots movement, but from a few very wealthy individuals with links to Big Ag and Big Pharma.

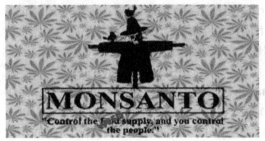

Leading the charge is George Soros, a major shareholder in Monsanto, the world's largest seed company and producer of genetically modified seeds. Monsanto is the biotech giant that brought you Agent Orange, DDT, PCBs, dioxin-based pesticides, aspartame, rBGH (genetically engineered bovine growth hormone), RoundUp (glyphosate) herbicides, and RoundUp Ready crops (seeds genetically engineered to withstand glyphosate).

Monsanto now appears to be developing genetically modified (GMO) forms of cannabis, with the intent of cornering the market with patented GMO seeds just as it did with GMO corn and GMO soybeans. For that, the plant would need to be legalized but still tightly enough controlled that it could be captured by big corporate interests. Competition could be suppressed by limiting access to homegrown marijuana; bringing production, sale and use within monitored and regulated industry guidelines; and legislating a definition of industrial hemp as a plant having such low psychoactivity that only GMO versions qualify. Those are the sorts of conditions that critics have found buried in the fine print of the latest initiatives for cannabis legalization.

Patients who use the cannabis plant in large quantities to heal serious diseases (e.g. by juicing it) find that the natural plant grown organically in sunlight is far more effective than hothouse plants or pharmaceutical cannabis derivatives. Letitia Pepper is a California attorney and activist who uses medical marijuana to control multiple sclerosis. As she puts it, if you don't have an irrevocable right to grow a natural, therapeutic herb in your backyard that a corporation able to afford high license fees can grow and sell to you at premium prices, isn't that still a war on people who use marijuana?

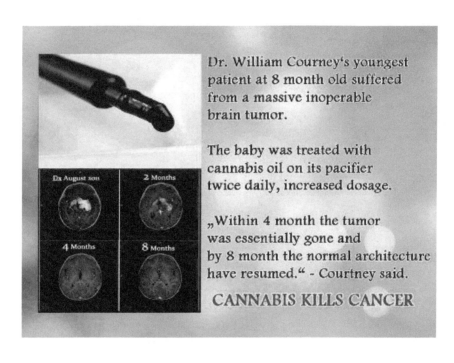

Dr. William Courney's youngest patient at 8 month old suffered from a massive inoperable brain tumor.

The baby was treated with cannabis oil on its pacifier twice daily, increased dosage.

„Within 4 month the tumor was essentially gone and by 8 month the normal architecture have resumed." - Courtney said.

CANNABIS KILLS CANCER

Chapter 8

Covidiocracy & the Really, Really Big Agenda

Ill-*HELL*th & Medi-*SINs*

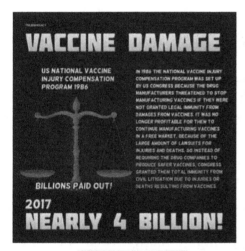
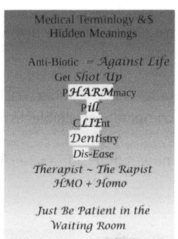
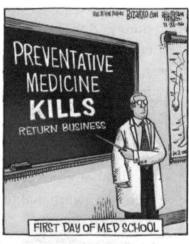

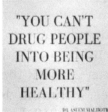
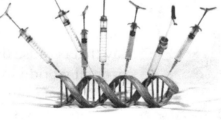
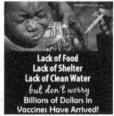

- The 3rd leading cause of death in humans is from hospitals!
- Western Medicine ranks *DEAD LAST in quality of care amongst 38 modern countries* and ranks #1 in cost, required coverage in many states
- Vaccines are now REQUIRED for all, with Zero Liability and only pure profits from the government paying for their products.
- We in the West die earlier and require more health 'care' than most other countries.

My medical father, when I asked him one day, "Dad, during your 30 years of medical *'practicing'* did you ever try to prevent people from getting sick… like eating healthier, yoga, meditation, etc."? His reply was quick and typical of the Western medical world, he said without any forethought, "Why would I want to do that? Because I'd be out of job and you never would of gotten into college, son, so be grateful!".

- Are you aware that western medical doctors can make an additional tens of thousands of dollars in 'performance bonuses' if they meet quotas to administer vaccinates set up by BigHARMa? Sometimes this amounts to double what they are being paid as doctors now in major hospitals!
- Are you aware doctors get paid to list the death of a patient as covid even if it was not the main cause of death?
- Are you aware western medical doctors cannot even promote self-breast examinations and that medical drugs cost multiple times more than the same drug in other countries, by design?
- Are you aware the CDC owns over 40 vaccine patents and profits from vaccine sales in the tens to hundreds of millions of dollars each year?
- Are you aware no drug companies are liable, in any way, for any injuries or illness' resulting from vaccines?
- Are you aware that it is now required in many states that we must carry the worst medical care possible by state law and show proof?
- Are you aware that forcing vaccines on people that are perfectly healthy is a crime against humanity?

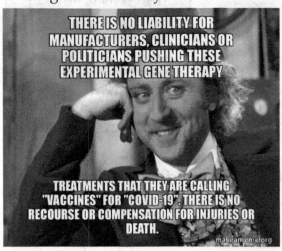

The Covid "Plannedemic", was designed and implemented as a bioweapon, not a cure for a totally fabricated and made up disease. I say that because the number of deaths in 2020 over all worldwide was LOWER than in 2019 and 2018 and Flu cases, including death…, in 2020 were **down 93% from 2019**. Even though few got flu shots in 2020! They have never had successful vaccines for even the common cold of flu for over 20 years and vaccine injuries have resulted in the US government paying out close to $4.5 BILLION in vaccine injuries to date, even though **BigHARMa is not liable in anyway** and doctors receive heavy bonuses for making their vaccine quotas, to name a few reasons.

It takes up to 10 years to create, and test, a new vaccine, yet Covid was given "emergency approval" without standard protocol testing. The initial testing done on ferrets killed them all when given the vaxxines. They simply halted the trials and rolled out 'the cure' and 'the prevention'. Now, more are getting ill, and *dying, from the vaxxines*! Biomagnetic protocols can address vaxxines injuries and issues like deactivating microchips and disallowing communications between chips and the mother ship collecting and controlling the data inside of us through 5G and other means.

Official Death Statistics as reported state by state for all of 2020 regarding death from Covid. **That is because there is no virus, PEOPLE ARE DYING FROM THE VAXXINE**, not the faux virus!!!

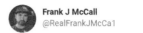
Just a reminder that Common flu cases dropped 99.99% last year

Frank J McCall
@RealFrankJMcCa1

It baffles me that the entire country does not question this.

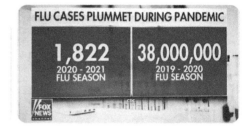

The Really Really Big Agenda

Magnetically Charged Nano Sized Robots in Vaxxines

This is from the National Institute of Health's website :

"Magnetogenetics is a new field that leverages genetically encoded proteins and protein assemblies that are sensitive to magnetic fields to study and manipulate cell behavior. Theoretical studies show that many proposed magnetogenetic proteins do not contain enough iron to generate substantial magnetic forces. Here, we have engineered a genetically encoded ferritin-containing protein crystal that grows inside mammalian cells. Each of these crystals contains more than 10 million ferritin subunits and is capable of mineralizing substantial amounts of iron. When isolated from cells and loaded with iron in vitro, these crystals generate magnetic forces that are 9 orders of magnitude larger than the forces from the single ferritin cages used in previous studies. These protein crystals are attracted to an applied magnetic field and move toward magnets even when internalized into cells. While additional studies are needed to realize the full potential of magnetogenetics, these results demonstrate the feasibility of engineering protein assemblies for magnetic sensing. NIH. gov*Engineering a Genetically Encoded Magnetic Protein Crystal*

You have seen the countless videos of magnets sticking to people after getting vaxxed and jabbed, now you know why and what they the nanobots being installed to override humans basic life operation systems!

Below are actual images of a 60 nanometer chip from the tip of test jab used for Covid testing. ***There can be up to 1 million nanobot chips in each vaxxines given as well is in the testing kits and swabs***. Once these chips are introduced to your system, they are said to be permanent and irreversible according to the manufactures.

State/Territory	Population	Total Cases	Total Death	Percentages Cases	Deaths	Odds of Surviving COVID-19
New York	19,450,000	343,705	27,284	1.767%	0.140%	99.860%
New Jersey	8,882,000	140,743	9,508	1.585%	0.107%	99.893%
Illinois	12,670,000	83,168	3,617	0.656%	0.029%	99.971%
Massachesets	6,893,000	79,332	5,141	1.151%	0.075%	99.925%
California	39,510,000	71,171	2,902	0.180%	0.007%	99.993%
Pennsylvania	12,800,000	61,407	3,924	0.480%	0.031%	99.969%
Michigan	9,987,000	47,946	4,674	0.480%	0.047%	99.953%
Texas	29,000,000	42,397	1,169	0.146%	0.004%	99.996%
Florida	21,480,000	41,915	1,778	0.195%	0.008%	99.992%
Maryland	6,046,000	34,927	1,809	0.578%	0.030%	99.970%
Connecticut	3,565,000	34,333	3,041	0.963%	0.085%	99.915%
Georgia	10,620,000	33,616	1,470	0.317%	0.014%	99.986%
Louisiana	4,649,000	32,050	2,281	0.689%	0.049%	99.951%
Virginia	8,536,000	32,050	2,281	0.375%	0.027%	99.973%
Indiana	6,732,000	25,676	1,578	0.381%	0.023%	99.977%
Ohio	11,690,000	25,257	1,436	0.216%	0.012%	99.988%
Colorado	5,759,000	20,103	1,009	0.349%	0.018%	99.982%
Washington	7,615,000	18,503	972	0.243%	0.013%	99.987%
North Carolina	10,490,000	15,832	614	0.151%	0.006%	99.994%
Tennessee	6,829,000	15,777	264	0.231%	0.004%	99.996%
Iowa	3,155,000	12,912	289	0.409%	0.009%	99.991%
Minnesota	5,640,000	12,494	614	0.222%	0.011%	99.989%
Arizona	7,279,000	11,736	562	0.161%	0.008%	99.992%
Rhode Island	1,059,000	11,614	444	1.097%	0.042%	99.958%
Wisconsin	5,822,000	10,625	418	0.182%	0.007%	99.993%
Alabama	4,903,000	10,494	442	0.214%	0.009%	99.991%
Missouri	6,137,000	10,125	530	0.165%	0.009%	99.991%
Mississippi	2,976,000	9,908	457	0.333%	0.015%	99.985%
Nebraska	1,934,000	8,734	103	0.452%	0.005%	99.995%
South Carolina	5,149,000	7,927	355	0.154%	0.007%	99.993%
Kansas	2,913,000	7,393	187	0.254%	0.006%	99.994%
Kentucky	4,468,000	7,003	157	0.157%	0.004%	99.996%
Delaware	973,764	6,741	237	0.692%	0.024%	99.976%
Washington DC	702,455	6,584	350	0.937%	0.050%	99.950%
Utah	3,206,000	6,454	73	0.201%	0.002%	99.998%
Nevada	3,080,000	6,311	321	0.205%	0.010%	99.990%
New Mexico	2,097,000	5,212	219	0.249%	0.010%	99.990%
Oklahoma	3,957,000	4,731	278	0.120%	0.007%	99.993%
Arkansas	3,018,000	4,164	95	0.138%	0.003%	99.997%
South Dakota	884,659	3,663	39	0.414%	0.004%	99.996%
Oregon	4,218,000	3,359	130	0.080%	0.003%	99.997%
New Hampshire	1,360,000	3,239	142	0.238%	0.010%	99.990%
Puerto Rico	3,194,000	2,329	115	0.073%	0.004%	99.996%
Idaho	1,787,000	2,294	69	0.128%	0.004%	99.996%
North Dakota	762,062	1,571	38	0.206%	0.005%	99.995%
Maine	1,344,000	1,477	65	0.110%	0.005%	99.995%
West Virginia	1,792,000	1,398	58	0.078%	0.003%	99.997%
Guam	165,768	1,121	6	0.676%	0.004%	99.996%
Vermont	623,989	929	53	0.149%	0.008%	99.992%
Wyoming	578,759	675	7	0.117%	0.001%	99.999%
Hawaii	1,416,000	624	17	0.044%	0.001%	99.999%
Montana	1,069,000	461	16	0.043%	0.001%	99.999%
Alaska	731,545	383	8	0.052%	0.001%	99.999%
U.S. Virgin Islands	106,977	69	6	0.064%	0.006%	99.994%
Northern Mariana Islands	56,882	19	2	0.033%	0.004%	99.996%

Nation & Territories	Population	Total Cases	Total Deaths	Overall Percentages Cases	Deaths	Odds of Surviving COVID-19
United States and it's territorie	331,762,860	########	83,654	0.417%	0.025%	99.975%

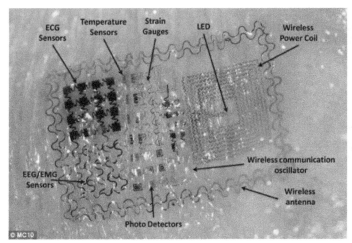

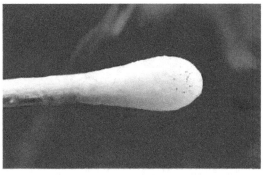

A theragripper is about the size of a speck of dust. This swab contains dozens of the tiny devices. Credit: Johns Hopkins University.

Inspired by a parasitic worm that digs its sharp teeth into its host's intestines, Johns Hopkins researchers have designed tiny, star-shaped microdevices that can latch onto intestinal mucosa and release drugs into the body.

There are over 500 more GMO vaxxines in the pipeline to come. The good news is that we can scan and find placements to help arrest, mitigate and possibly, eliminate the nanobots that come with the jab and the injections, yet all vaxxines are different from one another by design, so they will not have the same symptomology.

The goal of the world elite powers is to get everyone linked permanently to the cloud in what they call the IoT2IoB, or the Internet of Things connected to the Internet of Bodies. Our minds and bodies will be connected to the "cloud" where AI will own and control all. Magnetic nanoparticles (MNPs) are a class of engineered particulate materials of <100nm that can be manipulated under the influence of an external magnetic field.

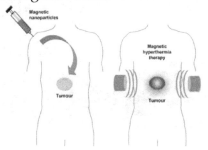

For a few decades, growing development in chemical synthesis of nanomaterials and material surface modification have been seen and performed in numerous applications including biomedicine, biotechnology, catalysis, magnetic chemistry thermoelectric materials, etc. Various methods for fabrication of MNPs which have a controllable size, distribution, and surface modification have been reported. In these methods, several techniques containing irradiation, microwave, ultrasonication, vapor deposition, electrochemical, and microwave are applied to produce MNPs either in bottom-up or top-down processes. Generally, magnetic synthesis of nanoparticles is carried out by using these two processes. Nanomaterials with magnetic properties have wide applications in many fields such as biology, medicine, and engineering. In this section, the recent developments in the structures, occurrences, most commonly used samples, and common areas of use of the MNPs are given.

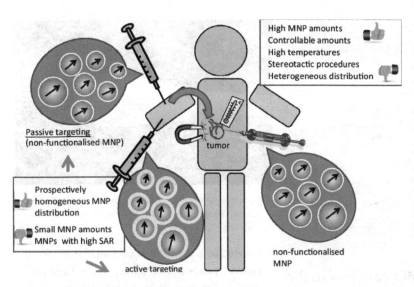

Magnetogenetics is the connecting nanomachinery they are using as shown in the diagram below. The good news is that we may be able to interrupt and/or disconnect the communication magneto's that interact with the 5G and 6G controlling mechanisms. A modified protein allows researchers to use a magnet to switch on neurons anywhere in the brain in freely moving mice and zebrafish. The tool, described in May in *Nature Neuroscience*, could shed light on neural circuits underlying autism-like behaviors in animal models of the condition Scientists can already turn neurons on and off at will with a technique called optogenetics that renders the cells sensitive to light. But that method requires surgically implanting a light source near the cells they want to manipulate. The researchers rendered an ion channel in neurons called TPRV4 magnetically sensitive by fusing it to ferritin, a protein rich in iron. TPRV4 is ordinarily heat- and pressure-sensitive, but the researchers reasoned that, when attached to ferritin, it would also open in the presence of a magnetic field. Opening the channel causes calcium to flow into the cell, prompting it to fire. Placing a magnet near cultured kidney cells expressing the protein, dubbed 'Magneto,' causes a calcium-sensitive fluorescent probe inside them

925 million 🖊 doses have now been administered worldwide

Totally unrelated photo:

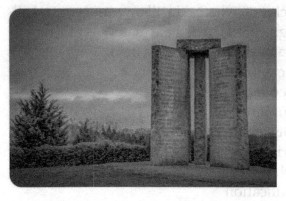

to light up within seconds. And placing a magnet next to brain slices from mice that had been 'infected' by a virus carrying the Magneto gene causes neurons in the slices to fire. This firing stops when the tissue is bathed in a drug that blocks TPRV4.

This proves that magnets can be used to harm and control or to heal and free and has been a part of overall healing for decades. If magnets were used to heal, we would all be living much longer, healthier lives, yet our winner take all system benefits those who can control all, including depopulation. In the Moderna Covid vaxxines includes a protein spike called SIM-102, polyethylene glycol [PEG] 2000 dimyristoyl glycerol [DMG], which is known to cause infertility! So why would they put this in the vaccines and then have mass reports of women getting irregular periods and men having infertility issues?

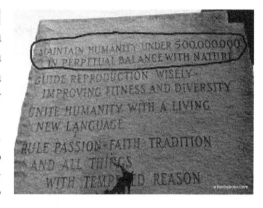

Google "Georgia Guidestones" to get your answer.

Again though, we can scan and find placements to help with infertility and such, so Biomagnetism may be critical to preserving life on Earth!... just imagine?

There has even been held a worldwide annual Biomag Conference on the many uses of magnets, which few are even aware of. This is because it works so well, costs little and everyone can benefit which totally goes against the capitalist capitalizing system of winner take all we have today.

The World Economic Forum (WEF) has unilaterally declared that humans will all become digitalized and own nothing by 2030 in their declared "4th Industrial Revolution" they have coined. There words:

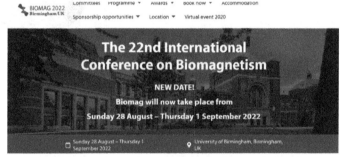

The Fourth Industrial Revolution represents a fundamental change in the way we live, work and relate to one another. It is a new chapter in human development, enabled by extraordinary technology advances commensurate with those of the first, second and third industrial revolutions. These advances are merging the physical, digital and biological worlds in ways that create both huge promise and potential peril. The speed, breadth and depth of this revolution is forcing us to rethink how countries develop, how organisations create value and even what it means to be human.

According to the projections of the WEF's "Global Future Councils," private property and privacy will be abolished during the next decade. The coming expropriation would go further than even the communist demand to abolish the property of production goods but leave space for private possessions. The WEF projection says that consumer goods, too, would be no longer private property. If the WEF projection should come true, people would have to rent and borrow their necessities from the state, which would be the sole proprietor of all goods. The supply of goods would be rationed in line with a social credit points system. Shopping in the traditional sense would disappear along with the private purchases of goods. Every personal move would be tracked electronically, and all production would be subject to the requirements of clean energy and a sustainable

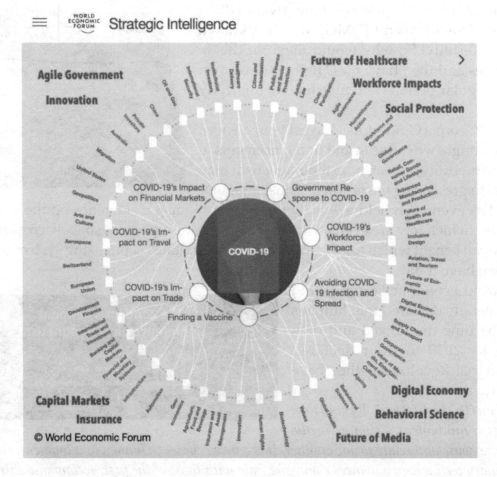

environment. In order to attain "sustainable agriculture," the food supply will be mainly vegetarian. In the new totalitarian service economy, the government will provide basic accommodation, food, and transport, while the rest must be lent from the state. The use of natural resources will be brought down to its minimum. In cooperation with the few key countries, a global agency would set the price of CO_2 **emissions** at an extremely high level to disincentivize its use.

In a promotional video, the World Economic Forum summarizes the eight predictions in the following statements:

1. People will own nothing. Goods are either free of charge or must be lent from the state.

2. The United States will no longer be the leading superpower, but a handful of countries will dominate.

Welcome To 2030: I Own Nothing, Have No Privacy And Life Has Never Been Better

World Economic Forum Contributor ⓘ
Leadership Strategy

By Ida Auken

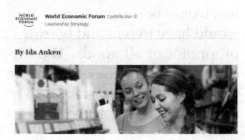

3. Organs will not be transplanted but printed.
4. Meat consumption will be minimized.
5. Massive displacement of people will take place with billions of refugees.
6. To limit the emission of carbon dioxide, a global price will be set at an exorbitant level.
7. People can prepare to go to Mars and start a journey to find alien life.
8. Western values will be tested to the breaking point..

Beyond Privacy and Property

In a publication for the World Economic Forum, the Danish ecoactivist **Ida Auken**, who had served as her country's minister of the environment from 2011 to 2014 and still is a member of the Danish Parliament (the Folketing), has elaborated a scenario of a world without privacy or property. In "**Welcome to 2030**," she envisions a world where "I own nothing, have no privacy, and life has never been better." By 2030, so says her scenario, shopping and owning have become obsolete, because everything that once was a product is now a service. In this idyllic new world of hers, people have free access to transportation, accommodation, food, "and all the things we need in our daily lives." As these things will become free of charge, "it ended up not making sense for us to own much." There would be no private ownership in houses nor would anyone pay rent, "because someone else is using our free space whenever we do not need it." A person's living room, for example, will be used for business meetings when one is absent. Concerns like "lifestyle diseases, climate change, the refugee crisis, environmental degradation, completely congested cities, water pollution, air pollution, social unrest and unemployment" are things of the past. The author predicts that people will be happy to enjoy such a good life that is so much better "than the path we were on, where it became so clear that we could not continue with the same model of growth."

Virus Spreading vs. Terrain Shedding ~ The Proof of Cover Up and Lies

Many people have heard the heartbreaking story about Nikola Tesla, and how Thomas Edison stole his work and caused him to go bankrupt. All the while Tesla has been pretty much erased from History Books...

But how many people know about Antoine Bechamp, and the massive fraud of a man that was Louis Pasteur? Not many I'd bet, as Bechamp was too erased from history. The reason behind this is actually much more sinister then one can imagine.

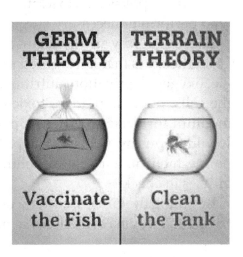

During his lifetime, Antoine Bechamp (1816-1908) was a well-known and widely respected professor, teacher, and researcher. He was an active member of the French Academy of Sciences, and gave many presentations there during his long career. He also published many papers, all of which still exist and are available.

And yet, he has disappeared from history.

On the other hand, Louis Pasteur (1822-1895) is one of the great rock stars of medicine and biology. Of the two – Bechamp or Pasteur – he's the one you've most likely heard of. His is one of the most recognizable names in modern science. Many discoveries and advances in medicine and microbiology are attributed to him, including vaccination and the centrepiece of his science – the germ theory of disease.

Louis Pasteur was actually a liar, a coward and a fraud. Pasteur renounced his own theory on his death bed. Germ Theory was all wrong: "*It's the terrain, not the germ.*" quoted Louis Pasteur on his death bed...

It's not the bacteria or the viruses themselves that produce the disease, it's the chemical by-products and constituents of these microorganisms enacting upon the unbalanced, malfunctioning cell metabolism of the human body that in actuality produce disease. If the body's cellular metabolism and pH is perfectly balanced or poised, it is susceptible to no illness or disease.

In other words, disease associated microorganisms do not originally produce a disease condition any more than a vulture produces a dead rabbit or rats produce garbage.

The diseased acidic cellular environment was created by a toxic diet, toxic environmental exposures and a toxic lifestyle supporting the morbid changes of germs to bacteria, bacteria to viruses, viruses to fungal forms and fungal forms to cancer cells in the body. This classical error of referring to symptoms as the disease is perpetrated to this day in all medical schools trickled down from the professors (whose bread is buttered by the pharmaceutical industry), to all med students with the intent of brainwashing the young, up and coming physicians to a kill mode mind-set and to be legal script writers and butchers who perform unnecessary surgical procedures.

The reason why all physicians are kept in the dark by medical schools teaching Pasteur's germ theory is that if they are taught the truth that it's the inner condition of the patient (i.e. oxygen deprivation, nutritional deficiencies, acidic pH, built up toxins in and around the cells, poor circulation, toxic emotions, etc.), not the germs that creates the growth medium for bacteria, viruses, parasites or cancer cell growth, the majority of doctors would throw away their script pad and surgical knife and focus their treatment protocols on reestablishing a healthy cellular environment, which keeps the germs, bacteria and viruses in check.

By killing the viruses, bacteria or cancer cells with their destructive weapons of war, they trigger microzyma evolution that makes the enemy pathogens stronger by creating resistant strains reaping more disease in the future. Nobody correlates their newly formed disease a year later with the past drug therapy. The result if the truth was told, a multi-billion dollar sick care industry that has been meticulously built by the global elite for a century would be exposed and crumble like the Babylonian empire of old. There is no medical doctrine so potentially dangerous as a partial truth implemented as whole truth.

Because of political reasons, Antoine Bechamp's name and research findings along with the germ theory controversy have been omitted from history, medical and biological books, even encyclopedias. It seems that the historical scientific assassination of Antoine Bechamp resulted in medical science's monopolization of pharmaceuticals and vaccine research. This has meant untold misery for the human race. It's ironic that Pasteur himself was reported to have admitted on his deathbed that Claude Bernard was right — the microbe is nothing, the terrain is everything, but would never give credit for Bechamp's discoveries. Bechamp's discovery in his early research, that all living things contain tiny granules, which he named microzyma's, was the most profound discovery of the 20th century.

Microzyma's can trigger life and/or Death. Microzyma's (meaning small ferments), inhabits cells, blood and lymph fluid. They act as both the builder and recycler of organisms. They inhabit cells, the fluid between cells, the blood and the lymph. In the state of healthy terrain. microzyma's act harmoniously and fermentation occurs normally and beneficially making healthy aerobic microbes like acidophilus and bifidus.

Under diseased pathological internal conditions (low oxygen, malnutrition, acidic pH, poor circulation, etc.), microzyma's can change the faces of microbes like a chameleon. This is called pleomorphism. Pleo means many and morph means form. So pleomorphism means to change to many forms. These pathogens can either evolve or devolve depending on the surrounding conditions of the cell. The answer in disease processes lies in the condition of your cellular balance or will it support the development of unwanted guests?

In the early stages of acidic pH in the body's tissues, the warning symptoms are mild. These include such things as skin eruptions, headaches, allergies, colds, flu and sinus problems. These symptoms are frequently treated (manipulated) with antibiotic drugs and suppressive medications. With continued suppression of the warning signals of an acidic and nutrient deficient environment, more serious symptoms arise with the disease driven deeper. Weakened organs and systems start to give way (heart, lung, thyroid, adrenals, the liver, kidneys, etc.).

Unfortunately, symptom manipulation with pharmacology creates a magical shell game of switching diseases, creating more serious symptoms and disease conditions in the future that are totally different from the original disease. The quick fix drug game of voodoo medicine is what's causing the disease epidemic in this country and puts hospitals and doctors as the number three killer in the U.S.

What is modern medicine doing with their destructive weapons of war? You can't kill microzymas, they're indestructible. You can only trigger a morbid evolution of anaerobic pathogens to molds, fungus, yeast and cancer. It's the microzymas that are responsible for the decomposition of a dead body back to the soil and creating life to the soil for future plant growth.

Microzymas are an indestructible living entity that cannot be destroyed by heat, antibiotics, or any other weapon of war. My view is that the toxins (acids) from the microforms combine to provoke the body to produce symptoms of a healing crisis to purge or eliminate the toxic residues from the nose through a runny nose, the skin through sweat, the colon through diarrhea, and increased respiration. So, it's important to remember, it is not the pathogens themselves which initiate disease, they only show up because of an acidic, compromised, cell terrain. Mosquitoes seek the stagnant water, but they don't cause the swamp to become stagnant.

All Disease Is Acid Related:

In general, degenerative diseases are the result of acid waste build-up within weak cells and organs that are too weak to clean house. When we are born, we have the highest alkaline mineral concentration, establishing the highest pH. That is why most degenerative diseases do not occur when you are young. They occur usually after 40 years of age.

The underlying causes of cancer, heart disease, arteriosclerosis, high blood pressure, diabetes, arthritis, gout, kidney disease, asthma, allergies, psoriasis and other skin disorders, indigestion, diarrhea, nausea, obesity, tooth and gum diseases, osteoporosis, morning sickness, eye diseases, etc., are the accumulation of acids in tissues and cells, poor blood and lymph circulation, and poor cell activity due to toxic acidic residues accumulating around the cell membrane which prevent nutritional elements from entering the cell.

All scavengers breed like parasites. After food is digested and absorbed into the bloodstream it is carried to *all 75 trillion cells of the body* via the circulatory system. The body eliminates what it can and the remainder settles in the weakest cells. Those which are not strong enough to clean house. In this accumulating, deposited, dead waste matter and pustulant soup, germs like bacteria, viruses, fungus and parasites breed. Rotting takes place and pus (which is decomposed blood), parasites, flukes, tapeworms, hardened mucous and other acid waste products form.

This, science calls disease:

The name of the particular disease depends upon the location of the deposits of this acidic, toxic, pustulant soup. If the accumulating deposits are in the joints, it's called arthritis. If the poisonous waste matter accumulates in the pancreas and saturates the beta cells that synthesize insulin it's called diabetes. If the toxic sludge is dumped in the lungs, it's called chronic obstructive pulmonary disease. It's the same disease. Wherever your weakest link in the chain of organs is, that's where your genetic disposition for disease will be.

If the overload is too great for the blood, excess acid is dumped into the tissues and cells for storage. Then the lymphatic system and immune system must neutralize what it can and attempt to discard the toxic waste. If the lymphatic system is overloaded generally due to a lack of exercise, acid deposits will suffocate the cells and damage DNA. If the lymphatic system is pumping through exercise and circulation, they will pick up the acid wastes and neutralize them through the kidneys. Unfortunately, they must dump them right back into the blood stream. This will force the blood to attempt to gather more alkaline salts in order to compensate while stressing the liver and kidneys. This robs Peter to pay Paul.

Body Electric

A healthy condition depends upon a high level of electromagnetic negative charge on the surfaces of tissue cells. Acidity is the opposite charge and dampens out these electrical fields. If tissue pH deviates too far to the acid side, cellular metabolism will cease and oxygen deprivation will occur. Acidity and lack of oxygen are the ideal environmental condition for morbid microforms to flourish. These are the primary symptoms of disease. So in short, acute or recurrent illnesses and infections are either the attempt by the body to mobilize mineral reserves from all parts of the body, or crisis attempts at detoxification. For example, the body may throw off acids through the skin, producing symptoms such as eczema, dermatitis, acne, or other skin disorders. Chronic symptoms result when all possibilities of neutralizing or eliminating acids have been exhausted. Unless the treatment actually removes acids from the body and replaces nutrient building blocks, the cure at best will be only temporary and a cover-up Band-Aid therapy, shoving the disease deeper into a chronic state. Remember, there is not one drug on the market that reduces the acidity of the body or addresses any kind of nutritional deficiency. The sobering fact is, almost all drugs are acidic, especially antibiotics, and add to the acid residues. And if the drugs were successful at removing acids from an infected area, the acid would migrate to some other weak tissue in the body that will create side effects there, unless the treatment involves the disposal of acids from all body organs. For this reason, today's medical science is pathetic when it comes to the cure for degenerative and metabolic disease.

Cancer Cell Growth Is Caused By Acid:

Let's look at cancer. If you were to ask an allopathic doctor to explain cancer in a few words, the best that they can come up with after all these years of research is a cell mutation, a missing gene, or maybe a virus causing immuno-suppression. Since cancer is not a localized disease, but a systemic condition, it shows up in the body's weakest link(s). I refer to the body's weakest links as the dead zones because they carry a declining electromagnetic charge. All healthy cells carry an electromagnetic negative charge, but all fermented cells and their acids carry an electromagnetic positive charge.

These rotting cells and their acids act like a glue (attracting each other) because opposites attract, causing healthy cells to stick together. This leads to oxygen deprivation where healthy cells begin to rot. This is cancer. It's my conclusion based on years of research and study that cancer and AIDS are nothing more or less than a cellular disturbance of the electromagnetic balance due to acid PH disorganization of the cellular microzymas, their morbid evolution to bacteria, yeast fungus and molds, and their production of exotoxins and mycotoxins. Cancer therefore is a four-letter word — ACID, especially lactic acid as a waste product due to the low oxygen level and waste products of yeast and fungus.

Dr. Otto Warburg, two time Nobel Prize winner, stated in his book, The Metabolism of Tumors. that the primary cause of cancer was the replacement of oxygen in the respiratory cell chemistry by the fermentation of sugar. The growth of cancer cells is initiated by a fermentation process, which can be triggered only in the absence of oxygen at the cell level. Just like over*worked muscle cells manufacture lactic acid by-products as waste, cancerous cells spill lactic acid and other acidic compounds causing acid pH.

If you cover your mouth, oxygen is cut off and carbon dioxide is built up as an acid waste and you will eventually pass out through asphyxiation. And if your body's blood pH goes below seven, oxygen is cut off and you will be put into a coma or death will occur. The blood performs a balancing act in order to maintain the blood pH within a safe range of 7.35 - 7.45. Some cells instead of dying as normal cells do in an acid environment may adapt and survive by becoming abnormal cells like primitive yeast cells. These abnormal primitive yeast cells are called malignant cells. Malignant renegade cells do not communicate with brain function, or with their own DNA memory code. Therefore, malignant cells grow indefinitely and without order. This biological disorder is what science calls cancer This could be improved by an alkaline diet and boosting the immune system.

During their lifetimes, the rivalry between Bechamp and Pasteur was constant, and often bitter. They clashed frequently both in speeches before the Academy, and in papers presented to it. Bechamp repeatedly showed that Pasteur's 'findings' included frequent plagiarizations (and distortions) of Bechamp's own work.

When Bechamp and others objected to the plagiarization, Pasteur set out to use his political clout to destroy Bechamp's career and reputation. Unfortunately, Pasteur largely succeeded. He was more skilful than Bechamp at playing politics and attending the right functions. He was good at making friends in high circles, and was popular with the royal family. Pasteur, in other words, was an A-lister. Bechamp was a worker.

The ideas, as well as the characters, of the two men were fundamentally opposed.

Pasteur argued for what we now call the 'germ theory' of disease, while Bechamp's work sought to confirm pleomorphism; the idea that all life is based on the forms that a certain class of organisms take during the various stages of their life-cycles.

This difference is fundamental. Bechamp believed that his work showed the connection between science and religion – the one a search after truth, and the other the effort to live up to individual belief. It is fitting that his book Les Mycrozymas culminates in the acclamation of God as the Supreme Source. Bechamp's teachings are in direct opposition to the materialistic views of the modern science of the twentieth century.

"These microorganisms (germs) feed upon the poisonous material which they find in the sick organism and prepare it for excretion. These tiny organisms are derived from still tinier organisms called microzyma. These microzyma are present in the tissues and blood of all living organisms where they remain normally quiescent and harmless. When the welfare of the human body is threatened by the presence of potentially harmful material, a transmutation takes place. The microzyma changes into a bacterium or virus which immediately goes to work to rid the body of this harmful material. When the bacteria or viruses have completed their task of consuming the harmful material, they automatically revert to the microzyma stage"

Mr. Antoine Bechamp was able to scientifically prove that germs are the chemical-by-products and constituents of pleomorphic microorganisms enacting upon the unbalanced, malfunctioning cell metabolism and dead tissue that actually produces dis-ease. Bechamp found that the diseased, acidic, low-oxygen cellular environment is created by a toxic/nutrient deficient diet, toxic emotions, and a toxic lifestyle. His findings demonstrate how cancer develops through the morbid changes of germs to bacteria, bacteria to viruses, viruses to fungal forms, and fungal forms to cancer cells. He found microzymas present in every cell in the bloodstream, in animals, in plants, and even in rocks. He found them present in the remains of dead animals many years after the animal's body had withered away to dust. He observed that in a healthy organism, microzymas work at repairing and nourishing all cells; but when the terrain becomes acidic, the microzymas morph into viruses, bacteria, yeast, fungus, and mold and prepare to break the host down.

Delta + Variant from India (Kamala) has now been named the #1 Variant in the US. Remember all the Indian symbolism in Pet Goat and Shiva doing her Death Dance? Delta Air based in Atlanta/Atlantis on the 33rd parallel, Home of the CDC, Ted Turner's Depopulation CNN, Georgia Guidestones, Walking Dead filmed, Race War MLK.

Alpha   Beta   Gamma   Delta

In genetics, it can stand for a gene deletion....
"(sign: Δ) is a mutation (a genetic aberration) in which a part of a chromosome or a sequence of DNA is left out during DNA replication. Any number of nucleotides can be deleted, from a single base to an entire piece of chromosome. The smallest single base deletion mutations occur by a single base flipping in the template DNA, followed by template DNA strand slippage, within the DNA polymerase active site.[2][3][4] Deletions can be caused by errors in chromosomal crossover during meiosis, which causes several serious genetic diseases. Deletions that do not occur in

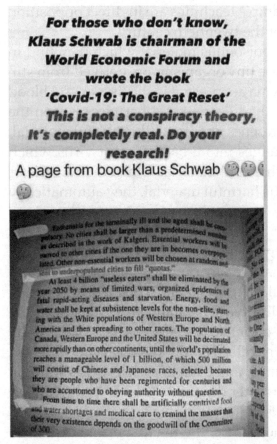

For those who don't know, Klaus Schwab is chairman of the World Economic Forum and wrote the book 'Covid-19: The Great Reset' This is not a conspiracy theory, It's completely real. Do your research!

A page from book Klaus Schwab 😐😐😐😐

multiples of three bases can cause a frameshift by changing the 3-nucleotide protein reading frame of the genetic sequence. Deletions are representative of eukaryotic organisms, including humans and not in prokaryotic organisms, such as bacteria. In genetics, a deletion (also called gene deletion, deficiency, or deletion mutation) (sign: Δ) is a mutation (a genetic aberration) in which a part of a chromosome or a sequence of DNA is left out during DNA replication. Any number of nucleotides can be deleted, from a single base to an entire piece of chromosome.

The Delta 32 gene Race Card?

Is this how they can delete certain races entirely as stated in Klaus "Darth" Schwab's book, "Covid-19: The Great Reset"? The intelligence agencies also prefer Rh negative people who possess the CCR5 Delta 32 gene, although this is not mandatory. The CCR5 delta 32 gene is a mutated form of the CCR5 gene. The Mutation is caused by a deletion of 32 base pairs normally found on the CCR5 gene. This gene is found only in European, West Asian and North African populations. The CCR5 delta 32 gene originated in the Caucasian race, and is only found in West Asian and North African populations due to admixture, and it isn't found in the Sub Saharan African population. This gene causes people to have a resistance to the HIV virus and other diseases that need the CCR5 protein to enter cells in order to cause infection.

Conclusion

Vibrational or energy medicine builds on the strengths of allopathic medicine and surgery in trying to do the best for our patients. There is a sound rationale and body of modern evidence that underpins an understanding of the subject but is not currently taught in medical or nursing

"Neurobiofeedback is emerging as a powerful tool in the rehabilitation of stroke patients."

Biofeedback Quote from the Desk of
Dr Sundardas D Annamalay
CEO, Sundardas Naturopathic Clinic

schools. Embracing new concepts, especially across disciplines, is always a challenge, especially at a time when much clinical and research practice appears to be ever more specialized.

Thus, concepts of "software" that are uncritically accepted if relating to the computer on our desks, can find great resistance in the biomedical fields, largely because the information is new and challenges tightly held and deeply cherished beliefs about the way the world and human beings are constructed. The irony is that we live our lives supported by material technology predicated upon microelectronic circuits fields, use text messaging, the World Wide Web and cloud computing, but we find difficulty in accepting that any of this might apply to our bodies or our beings.

If we concentrate only on allopathic approaches to disease, and look only at the physical, we may miss the point of health, life and living, and the British National Health Service will end up an unaffordable disease service – which is doomed to fail the unconscious and unarticulated health (mind, body and spirit) needs of its patients, despite ever more superb efforts by dedicated and expert technicians.

The answer? Education, education, education, inquiry and investigation at a personal level, to look at and examine these paradigms and attitudes, to recognize that we are each on a journey of learning in our lives, and to learn how to transform these paradigms and our own emotional and cultural baggage. Then, perhaps, we shall find how energy/ vibrational medicine can illuminate a way forward for us. Perhaps it is time to look at these paradigms and tendencies, to transcend them, and to find out interesting truths that have until now eluded us.

We are in the very first innings of a world healing protocol that, in time, may heal the whole world. We need specialists to focus on specific issues and symptoms, Biomag specialists in emotional placements, BiomagHospice and Biomag Pet care…..all needed

OPPORTUNITIES and Needs
Specialists Needed:

- Vets for the Pets
- Children:Autism, Vaccine injury, ADHD, etc.
- Elderly : Dimentia, Balance, Pain, Alzheimer,s etc.
- Insomnia: Brain Fog, Fatigue
- Infertility Menopause Sex Issues
  Pain: Arthritis, Shoulder, Knee, Inflamation
- Addiction; Alcohol, Buzz Kill
- Headaches
- Diet: Diabetes, Weight Loss
- Dentistry
- Sports Medicine
- Truamatic Brain Injury
- Skin Afflictions
- Chemtrails: Morgellons
- Jaramillo soup
  Magnetized Water, Refridgerators, Clothes (cooper bracelets)
- Making Magnets
- Lifestyle Change Coach
- Emotion: PTSD Grief Anger, etc.

possibilities in our headlights to come and learn and grow and heal. That is why I wrote this book so yu can learn and grow and share what has worked for you. Biomagnetism, and eventually hands-off healing, WILL heal this entire sickly world, once enough of us learn the World's Greatest Healing Protocol.

I am now two years on healing others, and myself, with magnets. Biomagnetism is evolving now into a full healing protocol that includes not just physical and emotional healing, but Spiritual healing/clearing as well. Mind, Body, Spirit. Thinking, Feeling, Willing. Will, Love and Wisdom. All part of the 3 part full healing protocol that is Biomagnetism. And, since magnets do not harm, anyone and everyone can learn to become effective healers in their own way, on their own terms, should they wish. This book was written with the intention to get the basics of magnetic healing to any and all who wish to learn and give a background outline as to how to conduct healing session with magnets. The more time you put into learning BMH protocol the more benefits you will derive, for yourself, and for you loved ones, including your pets.

Magnets are also excellent uses for addiction and detoxification. I have helped more than one with overcoming smoking, methane addiction and abuse of alcohol using Dr. Garcia's placements, as well as personal pairs for the individual. There is even protocols for immediately sobering up someone who has drunk too much by placing magnets on the kidneys and live. It is truly amazing to do the placements and watch the drunkard turn sober within 20 minutes and be able to drive home straight! More studies need to prove this out with breathalyzer testing and such.

The following appendixes are to be used to help scan and do placements. The sky is the limit as to how we can all learn this most amazing protocol and spread the news to others through empirical, and many times, immediate results that last.

Here's to healing the world...Hear! Hear!
Scan*Place*Heal

Appendix I

The Question Tree

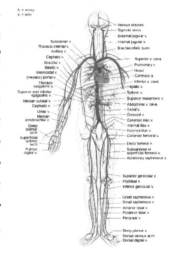

The healing comes from a level of everyone's highest poten-tial— that all encompassing, infinite, unbounded level of one's connection to their very existence. One does not have to travel anywhere to find That. It is already fully present with everyone. I use my intuition to 'feel' the presence of each person. Due to almost five decades of meditation, my access to Source is very smooth. My awareness acts as a bridge for everyone in the distance healing session. However, there is more. Once the bridge is formed, you don't need me anymore. I am only a temporary bridge until each person can access the infinite resource of their own Divine Being independently. I look forward to serving you.
~ **Dorothy Rowe**

Pre Exam

You may want to muscle scan for pH levels before the session. After, scan again to see if the pH levels have improved. This can be used as a baseline for your own proof that the session has been successful.

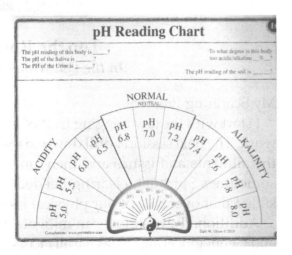

Reminders

Make sure the Soul you are facilitating is agree-able to change behaviors, diets, lifestyles, etc. that has caused the issues to arise. I also always ask is they wish to get healed when I begin the session work.

1. **Record Before and After**. Make sure to photograph/film any physical issues before session work begins so a before and after are proof of successful sessions!

2. **Manage Expectations**. Not everyone can be healed using magnets and some issues will take longer than other issues. Generally, the more serious issues, the more issues one has, the longer it can take to fully heal. Many sessions can be needed.

3. **Scan Dr. Garcia's Protocol Scan Sheet** first, including Most Common Pathogens (if you find Malaria, Tuberculosis, Epstein Barr Virus, Rabies, Psuedomona Auregonsa and/or Yersinia Pestis, then do all placements for that pathogen).

4. **Scan by Symptoms And Issues and Ailments**. (Note that body parts may have been removed, i.e. Thyroid take out, yet energetically placements may still be needed or asked for.)

5. **Scan by Emotions** as found or first or last

6. **Scan for Reservoir Clearing** to purge toxic cells broken up during session work.

7. **Scan Nutritional Charts** for Additional Supplements and Diets as well as Ch. 7.

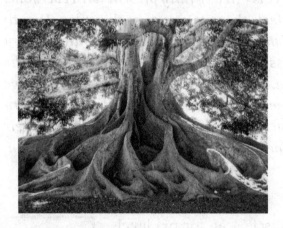

Too the Roots of the Problems
In the Questions You Will Find the Answer

My Scanning Protocol

I start with the low hanging fruit of issues the soul is experiencing with the first session work. The next session I drill down to the branch and trunk of the issues of what is causing the ailments and issues and then, on the 3rd session, I go deep into the emotional, and sometimes Spiritual, clearing needed for full recovery. Remember that Dr. Garcia has stated that over 80% of our physical issues are emotionally based.

Additionally, we know can mitigate effects of our toxic terrain from vaxxines, Pfoods, and Geonegineering issues we all face, so regular checkups and regularly interval scanning as follow up is suggested as well.

Before I even take on a soul to help facilitate their healing, I muscle test to ask this soul is someone I can help today? If yes, I accept the offer to help, if I muscle test and get a "no" response, I do not take on the session. However, their may be a time when you can help them in the future, so you can as that as well by muscle testing. Some souls are not ready to get healed, or they need to overcome other issues and experiences before they are "available" to be healed with magnets.

Soul Sessions

My general method for assisting healing for a Soul is to start with 3 sessions that can go for 45 minutes to several hours in more severe symptoms and issues. Sometimes 3 sessions, or even one session, can produce profound results.

Session 1 Fruitful — I focus on general clearing using Dr. Garcia's protocol scan sheet and the souls issues and symptoms they are experiencing. I call this the "fruit session" because I'm dealing with the low hang, surface issues that the soul is experiencing.

Session 2 Branches and Trunks — The next session I drill down into issues that reoccur from previous session as well as new findings and then drill down to find exactly where the toxic cells may be located.

Session 3 Roots — I get into emotional clearing as well as another over all scan. There are after every session I do Reservoir Clearing as my final placements, if needed. There are literally hundreds of emotions to scan for, as listed below. You can then ask "with this emotion, is their physical issues we can address with magnets"? If "yes" you would then scan for the correct placements.

Mindful Purpose

It is important to set your own intentions when beginning session work for a soul. What is your purpose today with this individual? Why are you here today for this soul session? What are your intentions to assist this soul? Do you have any expectations or desires of outcomes? Is your scanning biased at all by your feelings for this person?

Muscle testing will guide you through the entire healing protocol question tree presented here. Trust your muscle testing and go back again and confirm, confirm, confirm until you are satisfied, and muscle testing confirms, you have assisted this soul all you can with this session.

It is critically important that you ask permission and the abilities to conduct a soul session with that individual you wish to assist and help. Some are not ready to be healed and may have unresolved karma conflicts that need to still be experienced.

Sidebar: If everyone learns to muscle test then all will have in built in B.S. detectors! And everyone will *know* who is being deceitful and who is being honest and the world will be healed because all would now have to tell the truth or be outed by each individual! What a world it will be, indeed.

How Long to Leave Magnets On?

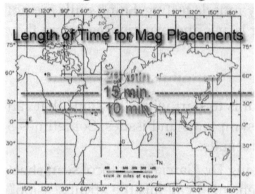

Your latitude where the soul resides will determine timing of how long to keep the magnets on the soul you are assisting since we are connecting with Earth's magnetic core.

If north of Mid USA latitudes place for 20 minutes, 15 minutes at SF-NY latitude and less if south of USA borders place for 10 minutes. It matters not if the magnets are left on too long, yet no benefit will be derived.

BE SPECIFIC and DIRECT with YOUR QUESTIONS

It is critical that the more specific your Yes/No question is, the more accurate response you will get. (i.e. What is wrong with this person? Vs. Are their issues here to deal with today in the head, neck, etc..? Is this placement correct? Does there need to be another placement associated? Do they need follow up placements? If so, when..??, etc., etc.)

To Spirit guide, "Will you allow me to help this soul **today**"? (Make sure to say "help them **today**". You may be able to assist them in the future and you wish to focus on today. If no, ask if there would be another time to assist? Days, weeks, etc?

My point of view is that I am a conduit for the Spirit being(s) to work through me so I also make sure I am healthy, mentally and physically and have a clear mind. A Biomag Healer should begin by asking what is there goals today? To alleviate pain, to find root causes, to deal with emotional issues.

These questions are in relation to whom you are working with, what are their immediate and long-term needs? How critical is the session? Will they want, be available for, follow up sessions? I start each session with a prayer of gratitude. This reminds me that I am not the healer. I am only the witness to the transformations which are orchestrated by the presence of God in each person. These healings occur through an activation of the body's own healing mechanisms.

In Person Session

In person sessions can last up to 2 hours or more in some cases, so make sure they are warm, comfortable and have gone to the bathroom first. I first do a "Chakra Clearing" to begin the session as to get their energy fields activated. You can see the placement chart below. What I have found this also does is in many cases, bring a physical sensation the soul that they can feel themselves, which helps validate the magnetic healing protocols as well as give them a positive 'vibe' that BiomagHealing works.

Another positive effect of the soul just thinking it may help them is called the "placebo effect". This has proven to occur up to 20% of the time, if the soul "believes" they will get better. The **placebo effect** is when an improvement of symptoms is observed, despite using a nonactive treatment. It's believed to occur due to **psychological** factors like expectations or classical conditioning. Research has found that the **placebo effect** can ease things like pain, fatigue, or depression.

Hands On Healing

1. Ask "Soul, do you wish to be helped with your issues today"? If yes, continue. If no, then you need to find out why. Remember, we are facilitators to their own healing.

2. "Soul, how much time do you have for the session today" in case you need to go deeper and want to know if you can facilitate more time.

3. "Soul, are you willing to change diet, lifestyle, etc. to heal yourself"? Listen carefully to their answer. If they waver at all, then they are not willing to do whatever is necessary to heal themselves, so ask them why?

In Person or Distance Healing

1. "Am I connected to this soul?" Ask at regular intervals during your session work. (Any breaks in focus, again ask if you are still connected to the soul you are assisting).

2. Command the body to speak to you about what it wants in order to heal. "I command you show me what placements this soul needs today".

Let's Begin

Intentional Healing and Scanning

Review muscle scanning techniques and become adept at receiving responses to get very comfortable with your muscle testing confirmation process. This video is a teach in for those wishing to learn different ways to muscle test.

https://youtu.be/YGRJoJMnuVc

Confirmation. Confirmation. Confirmation

Confirming your findings is critical. In that it assures you that you are correct and builds confidence in your placement protocols. I always, always ask the same? twice

1. Do I need another placement? No.

2. Are you sure? Yes.

(*This way you get your muscles to confirm, confirm, confirm with movement to ensure your muscle testing is still working properly.*)

There are as many ways to begin to scan someone as there are biomagnetic placements. The most effective, the most proven, is far and away Doctor Garcia's Beyond Biomag Healing Protocol scan sheet that allows for scanning the entire body from head, neck, thorax, abdomen, pelvis, post thorax (back), arm, lets and emotions to begin.

Or you can also begin with addressing specific issues (emotional, pain, inflammation, insomnia, etc.). This is what I call the "low hanging fruit" in that you can usually get immediate results and it helps alleviate physical issues, but does not get into the emotional, mental, or causal factors of what is the root of the cause.

As stated earlier, I start my first session looking at the tree of the soul, then the core causal issue, then the emotions and associated pairs. I call it *"Drilling Down to Find the Radical Root of the Problem"*. "Radical" means getting to the square root of the problem in mathematics.

A. Focus on specific issues (insomnia, pain, emotional issues, etc.)
B. Follow Dr Luis Garcia's Scan Sheet Protocol (recommended)
C. Scan Protocol: 1**) Head 2) Neck 3) Thorax 4) Abdomen 5) Pelvis 6) Back 7) Arms 8) Legs and 9) Emotions associated?**

Once you locate a placement. Then follow up and muscle test to ask:

1. Black on right or left side? Red on right or left side? (remember to reverse placement to what you see in the Bible)
2. Then muscle test to ask if each placement is correct? If not correct, ask should the placement be higher, lower, left or right?
3. Ask if more magnets are needed on this placement? You can just add magnets as needed, I've put up to 5 stacks of magnetic pairs at times as needed.
4. Ask is there are associated pairs with this issue?
5. If yes, find associated pairs by drilling down, is this in the vein, artery, nerves, bone, ligament, joint or space inbetween? I will bring up anatomy charts to better target the EXACT spot of placement of my intention with the magnets. Remember your intention is the power working with the magnets.
6. Keep repeating and repeating until you no longer get any placements needed. When you ask "Are there any more placements I need to help this soul with today"? an you get a "no" response, then your session work is conclude
7. Ask then, does this soul need a follow up session? And then scan for when..(day, weeks, etc.)

"How long do I leave the magnets on"? Set time of each placement with your intention. You can then muscle test and ask, "do I need more time on this placement"? If no, then you can remove the magnetic pairs.

Dr. Garcia's Protocol ~ Drilling Down Body Scan

Some placements are what are called "Personal Pairs". These are placements unique to each individual and may not be in the Biomag Practioners Guide aka BM Bible, so you must scan to find out where the magnets need to go for this individual. Once you locate where the black or red placement needs to go, I ask if this placement, be it a pair, or individual black or red placement, is it in the "Biomag Bible"? Is yes I follow Dr. Garcias protocol to locate placements needed, whether as a pair, or individually red or black. If no, I then ask for the specific placement in that area.

Body Scanning

Ask:

1. "Is this specific issue I am looking for placement in the **Head, Neck, Thorax, Abdomen, Pelvis, Arms, Legs,** or the **Posterior Thorax** (back)? (The Beyond Biomag Practitioner's guide flows this way.)

2. Is the correct placement for the "….." on this Protocol Scan Sheet? If no, then it is a specific placement for that soul. Find the placements by drilling down, "does the black go the head, neck, etc..and does the corresponding red placement go…?)

3. If you get a "Yes", (ex. In the Abdomen, "is it this one, this one…?") and go down the scan sheet.

After pair of placements ask:

A) Is this placement is correct?

B) Are more magnets needed?,

C) Are there associated placements needed?

Repeat. Repeat. Repeat.

Advanced Scanning

Dr. Garcia's session work lasts usually for 90 minutes and he will have placed over 30-40 pairs in that time. His scanning goes much deeper than what I described above. For example, he has a virus sheet of over 300 placements alone, as well as lists and lists of other pathogens so he can dial in EXACTLY where he underlying issues are. This is just an outline of further, deeper, more to the root scanning techniques. He has compiled these additional hundreds of placements over his 13 years of BiomagHealing.

Drilling Down to the Roots

1. Scan to Find and Issue and Location

2. Then ask is this issue we are focusing on located in the ?

   a. Arteria

b.   Vein

c.   Nerves

d.   Muscle

e.   Ligament

f.   Joint

g.   Space

3.   Once the specific are is located *you will need to look at an anatomy chart* of the nerve, vein, muscle, etc. identified and ask whether it is in the head, neck, thorax, pelvis, post thorax, arms, legs etc. These can be known common placements in Dr. Garcia's bible, but likely will be personal placements so you need to search for:

a.   where does the black placement go? And the red? Associated pairs?

b.   will they need follow up placements?

Finally, there are literally a million questions you can asks and verify with muscle testing to find the root of the issues and get effective results that are long lasting. In addition, asking again and again to get confirmation will solidify your validating placements and locations.

Basics Session Reminders

1.   Not everyone is ready to be healed through Biomagnetic Protocols

2.   Manage Expectations about what can and cannot be accomplished

3.   Over 80% of the time the placements are Black down on skin on the *Right Side* of the body and Red down on skin on *Left Side*. This is because most of us are heavily inbalanced to an acidic state and need to be much more alkalined to heal and prevent illness.

4.   The images in Dr. Garcia's Handbook are flipped over from image you see. (ex. If you see black over heart, put black Down for placement, not other side of the body)

5.   Remember to flush with Reservoir clearing when finished.

6.   Remember to give thanks for Spirit Beings helping guide you in this healing process.

7.   Make sure to muscle test to make sure you remain connected to the soul you are helping facilitate their healing.

8.   If remote healing, set timing lengths for placement of magnets.

9.   Ask if the soul can help themselves with placing magnets themselves? Show them where and how to put the placements.

10. Give the soul suggestions as to what they can do (change diet, meditate, stop eating dairy, etc.) to help facilitate their healing.

Conclusion of Session and Follow Up

1. Does soul need a follow up session with me?
2. When? In 1 day, 1 week, 1 month, etc.?
3. How many more sessions will they need?

Suggest them to drink plenty of water and that they may have Herxheimer issues. A Herxheimer reaction is when the body goes to clear itself of toxic issues released by the healing session. This can last a day or two, yet reservoir clearing will mitigate much of these reactions. It is like someone working out for the first time in a while. Their muscles first, get sore, then the muscles adapt and strengthen, same principles.

Make sure they can contact you with any follow up questions or issues they may be having after the session.

MAKE SURE TO DOCUMENT BEFORE AND AFTER session work. Many forget how ill they were when they begin to feel better and you will be building a book of testimonials for your business and to share with others.

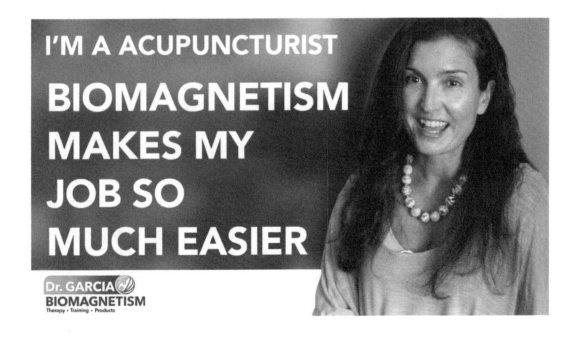

Appendix II

Scan Charts and Session Protocols

R eservoir clearing should be done at the beginning and at the conclusion of each session. As toxic cells are broken up, they are then broken up once more by the final reservoir clearing, thereby being now fuel for the health cells to consume and to mitigate Herxheimers effects.

You will need the Biomag Practioners Guide Handbook to look up page numbers from scan sheets below. This book contains over 300 placements and can be purchased at Usbiomag.com/ products.

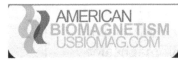

The following images are taken from Dr. Garcia's Biomag "Bible" and is an essential guide for Biomag Healing. You can order the book at usbiomag.com.

The 1st column are the placements, black first, then red placements (but muscle test each time).

The 2th column symbolism; R = Reservoir, B = Bacteria, P = Parasite, F = Fungus and V = Virus. SP = Special Pairs, PP = Personal Pairs, DP = Dysfunctional Pairs and E = Emotions.

The 3rd column "interpretation" is Doc G's notations on issues. When I find the placement called for, I then muscle test the interpretations to see if any of these apply ot the soul I am facilitating.

The 4th column is the page number in the Beyond Biomagnetism Practitioners Guide to find the correct placements.

When I scan these protocol pages I ask "Are their placements on this page I need to look at"? If I get a "yes" I scan the page. If "no", I go to the next page. When I finish the all the scan sheets I ask, "Do I need to go back over the scans sheets again"? The reason we do this is that we are like peeling on onion, layers on layers of issues that can be revealed once other issues are addressed.

The more you keep asking, "Do I need to look further", the better your success rate will be. Drill, drill, drill until you get an "all done" for that session.

Note: These are the most common pathogens Dr. Garcia has found and should be a primary scan in every session. (See next page) If you find any issues while scanning with Yersinia Pestis, Malaria, Rabies, Psuedomonia Aeruginosa and Epstein Barr Virus (EBV), ALL placements are needed in the box where the issue was found.

I have also broken down the Bible onto and Excel spread-sheets to be able to quickly scan for issues, symptoms, and ailments specifi-cally. If you wish a copy, after you have purchased the Bible, send me an email at Biomaghealer@ gmail.com and I will send the link to you.

Dr Garcia Most Common Pathogens 2020

Yersinia species

1	Vagina	Vagina Horizontal
2	Testicle	Testicle
3	Lung (Left Top)	Lung (Left Bottom)(Vertical)
4	Thyroid	Thymus
5	Spleen	Spleen (Vertical) (Mycoplasma)
6	Duodenum	Spleen
7	Transverse Colon	Vagina/Testicle (Left)
8	Lung(Left)	Vagina/Testicle (Left)
9	Bladder	Vagina / Left Testicle (Reservoir)
10	Vagina	Throat (Yersinia PseudoTB)

Rabies Virus

1	Armpit	Armpit
2	4th Rib	4th Rib (Dr. G)
3	Peri-Pancreatic	Peri-Pancreatic (Vertical)
4	Sphincter of Urethra	Sphincter of Urethra (Horizontal)

Mycobacterium Tuberculosis

1	Spleen	Left Lung
2	Corpus Callosum Center	Corpus Callosum Left Border
3	Spermatic chord	Spermatic chord
4	Supraspinatus	Supraspinatus
5	Fibula Head	Fibula Head
6	Right Lung	Left Lung
7	Bladder	Vagina (Resevoir)

Immune Stimulation & Gut

1	Thymus	Rectum (HIV)
2	Renal Capsule Left	Left Kidney
3	Adductor	Adductor
4	Triceps	Triceps
5	Bladder	Vagina
6	Appendix	Thymus

Pseudomona aeruginosa

1	Pleura (Left Top)	Pleura (Left Bottom) (Mycoplasma)
2	Thyroid	Liver
3	Adrenals	Lung (Left)
4	Pubic bone	Pubic bone
5	Rectum	Rectum (Horizontal)

Epstein Barr Virus (EBV)

1	Occipital	Occipital
2	Pleura Left	Lung (Left)
3	Sternocleidomastoides Left	Thymus
4	Heel Right	Heel Left
5	Roof of right eye	Roof of left eye

Lyme Co-Infections

1	Borrelia (Costal Liver/Liver)	Babesia
2	Bartonella	Theileria
3	Rickettsia (Temporal[2] / Wrists[1] / Calcaneus[2])	Mycoplasma (Pectoralis[2] / Temporal-Occipital[2])
4	Tularemia (Thymus/Pineal)	Ehrlichia
5	Tuberculosis (7 pairs)	Coxiella
6	Yersinia (8 Pairs)	Anaplasma
7	Epstein Barr Virus (5 pairs)	CMV (R. Eye/L. Eye)
8	Malaria (10 pairs)	Rabies (4 pairs)

SPECIAL Pairs

Co-infections	Dairy
Hepatitis	Emotions
Mosquitos	Lyme Other

Malaria (Plasmodium species)

1	Cheek	Contralateral Kidney
2	Cervical 1	Pylorus
3	Cervical 3	Bladder
4	Left Carina	Bladder
5	Palm	Palm
6	Clavicle	Clavicle
7	Head of Pancreas	Bladder
8	Bladder	5th Lumbar
9	Bladder	Left Kidney
10	Bladder	Vagina (Resevoir)

Pathogenic Virus

1	Cytomegalovirus (CMV)(Eye/Eye)	Encephalitis V (Parietal[2])
2	Aftosa Virus (Carina[2]), Thoracic Vert.3 / Thoracic Vertabrea 7	Guillan Barre V. (Pineal / Medulla, Pylorus/Medulla)
3	Zika (Ant. Costal (L)/Left Kidney)	Newcastle (Medulla/Cerebellum)
4	Dengue V. (Pituitary/Bladder), Medulla/Bladder	Coxsackie (Sternum Manubrium[2])
5	Rotavirus (Coccyx/Coccyx, Spleen/Adrenal)	HTLV (Suprapubic[2]), Inguinal Nerve[2]
6	HERV(Human Endog. RetroVirus)	HERPES Family of Virus
7	Respiratory Syncitial Virus (Frontal Sinus[2], Eyebrow[2], Paranasal Sinus[2])	HPV (Anus[1], Prostate/Rectum or Anus)

Pathogenic Bacteria

1	Proteus (Mediastinum[2], Costal[2], Renal Capsule[2], Sacrum[2], Body of fibula[2])	Cholera (Transverse Colon/Bladder, Transverse Colon/Liver)
2	Clostridium (Botulinum, Dificile, Tetanicum, Perfringens, Malignum)	Treponema palidum (Deltoid Tuberosity[2], Quadratus Lumborum[2])
3	H.pylori (Hiatus/Right Testicle)	Chlamydia Species
4	Neisseria Gonorrhea (Inframental tubercule/ Gonion Left), Lumbar 4[2]	Mycobact. Lepra (Scapula[2])
5	Legionella (Thymus/Cardiac Sphincter, Acromiom[2], T2[2])	Brucela (Liver/Spleen, Spleen/Liver, Diaphragm/Left Kidney
6	Staphyloccocus species	Streptococcus species
7	Anthrax (Craneal[2])	E. coli

VACCINES

1	English Measles (Rubeola)	Mumps
2	German Measles (Rubella) (Thymus/Parietal lobe Left, A/V Node / Left Kidney)	Rotavirus (Coccyx/Coccyx, Spleen/Adrenal)
3	Hepatitis A	Hepatitis B (Right Pleura / Liver)
4	Diphtheria	Tetanus (Kidney/Kidney)
5	Pertussis	Pneumococcal polysaccharide
6	Typhoid	Haemophilus Influ B (HIB)
7	Poliovirus (T10/T10, Sciatic Nerve[2])	Human Papilloma Virus (HPV)
8	Varicella	Meningitis (Medulla/Thyroid)
9	Varicella Zoster Ascending C/ Descending Colon)	Smallpox (Appendix/Left Tongue)
10	Yellow Fever	Adenovirus

Pathogenic Fungus

1	Candida	Aspergillus
2	Histoplasma	Cryptococcus
3	Pneumocystis	Stachybotrys
4	Trycophytum	Mucormycosis
5	Mycetoma	Ringworm
6	CDC website: Other	Talaromycosis

Pathogenic Parasites

1	Mites / Scabies	Zoonotic Infections
2	Tapeworm	Protozoa
3	Hookworms	Entamoeba species
4	Fluke	Giardia
5	Pinworm	Endolimax
6	Roundworms	Cysticercosis
7	Anisakis	Trichomonas
8	Other Parasite	Blastocystis hominis

www.usbiomag.com

Dr. Garcia's Biomagnetism Scan Sheet

Name:

Issues:

Age: **Foreign DNA:**   **Other:**   **Date:** DD MM YYYY

R = Reservoir, B = Bacteria, V = Virus, P = Parasite, F = Fungus, S = Special, D = Dysfunction, T = Trauma, E = Emotional

				S#1	S#2	S#3	INTERPRETATION	PAGE
RESERVOIRS								
1	KIDNEY/BLADDER (Other)	PAIN	R				Infection, wound, bum, muscle contractures	31
2	STUMP/SCAR	STUMP/SCAR	R				Scars	31
3	TOOTH	KIDNEY (homolateral)	R				Infection in tooth, gum, or alveolar bone	32
4	BLADDER	TOOTH	R				Infection in tooth, gum, or alveolar bone	32
5	NUTRIENT ARTERY	NUTRIENT ARTERY	R				Universal reservoir	33
6	PELVIC FLOOR	PELVIC FLOOR	R				Mainly bacteria reservoir, menstrual cramps, bloating	33
7	APPENDIX	BLADDER	R				Bacterial reservoir	34
8	SCAPULA	SCAPULA	B				Immune stimulation, cancer, eye isues, dry nasal membrane	34
9	RENAL CAPSULE	KIDNEY	R				Stimulates and restores kidney function, HIV	35
10	GALLBLADDER	GALLBLADDER	R				HIV, Hep B	35
11	CARDIAC SPHINCTER	TEMPORAL (L)	R				Vaccines, dementia, uncontrolled muscle movements	36
12	URETHRA	URETHRA	R				Universal reservoir	36
13	INTERILIAC	SACRUM	R				Parasite reservoir, can cause retention of toxins	37
14	FEMORAL NECK	FEMORAL NECK	R				Fungus reservoir, osteoperosis	37
HEAD								
15	POSTPOLE	POSTPOLE	B				Equilibrium, confusion, headaches, psychological disorders	39
16	POLE	POLE	S				Verical equilibrium, dyslexia, stuttering, learning disorders	39
17	PITUITARY	PITUITARY	D				Endocrine disorders, stimulates gastrointestinal tract and thyroid	40
18	PITUITARY	MEDULLA	S				Diabetes, metabolic disorder, lg. amts of dilute urine, dehydration	40

236

Dr. Garcia's Biomagnetism Scan Sheet

R = Reservoir, B = Bacteria, V = Virus, P = Parasite, F = Fungus, S = Special, D = Dysfunction, T = Trauma, E = Emotional

				S # 1	S # 2	S # 3	INTERPRETATION	PAGE
19	PITUITARY	OVARY	S				PMS, malnutrition, postpartum, pituitary issues, pelvic infections	41
20	PITUITARY	BLADDER	V				Dengue, vomiting, diarrhea, common cold symptoms	41
21	FRONTAL SINUS	FRONTAL SINUS	V				Abundant mucus, common cold, headaches, fevers with chills	42
22	GLABELLA	MEDULLA	S				Self-esteem, body issues, psychological trauma, abortions	42
23	INTERCILIARY	MEDULLA	S				Overbearing character, excessive shyness, insecurities, phobias	43
24	CRANIAL	CRANIAL	B				Abundant mucus, headaches, flu-like symptoms, visual symptoms	43
25	LACRIMAL DUCT	LACRIMAL DUCT	B				Nose bleeds, rhinitis and laryngitis, barky cough and hoarse voice	44
26	EYEBROW	EYEBROW	V				Congestion, respiratory infections, anxiety, irritability, tremors	44
27	EYELID	EYELID	B				Conjunctivitis, sinusitis, otitis media, laryngitis, bronchitis	45
28	EYE	EYE	V				Deformation of retina, cataract, eye pain, fatigue, MS	45
29	EYE	CEREBELLUM	S				Inflammation of optic nerve, ocular surgeries	46
30	ORBITAL FLOOR	ORBITAL FLOOR	V				Macular degeneration, keratoconus, affects retina	46
31	CANTHUS LATERAL	CANTHUS LATERAL	F				Black mold in vegetables, glaucoma, fungus in environment	47
32	TEMPLE	TEMPLE	S				Improves cerebral and pulmonary circulation, headaches.	47
33	CHIASM	CHIASM	S				Regulates lymphatic system, edemas in arms and legs, eyestrain	48
34	CIRCLE OF WILLIS	CIRCLE OF WILLIS	V				Smallpox, insomnia, dementia, brain fog	48
35	CHEEKBONE (L)	KIDNEY (R)	P				Malaria, fevers, chills, confusion, headaches, vomiting	49
36	MALAR	MALAR	V				Diarrhea, headaches, flu-like symptoms, abdominal pains, vomiting	50
37	ETHMOID/SPHENOID	ETHMOID/SPHENOID	R				Sinus, runny nose , headache, ear pressure, loss of smell, bad breath	50
38	NOSE	NOSE	S				Inhalation of mold or chemicals, snorting drugs, prescription meds	51
39	MAXILLARY SINUS	MAXILLARY SINUS	V				Sinusitis, headaches, stuffy nose, mouth breathing	51
40	MAXILLA	MAXILLA	B				Thick mucus with foul odor, urinary tract infection, pneumonia	52
41	COMMISSURE	COMMISSURE	V				Herpes, mucus in mouth and cheeks, mouth cancer	52
42	TONGUE	TONGUE	P				Blisters and itching, hair loss, transmitted by animal hair	53

Dr. Garcia's Biomagnetism Scan Sheet

R = Reservoir, B = Bacteria, V = Virus, P = Parasite, F = Fungus, S = Special, D = Dysfunction, T = Trauma, E = Emotional

			S #1	S #2	S #3	INTERPRETATION	PAGE
43	PREAURICULAR	PREAURICULAR	B				Nocardia, cough, shortness of breath, fever	54
44	PAROTID	PAROTID	D, V				Weight loss, digestive disorders, calcium deficiencies, mumps (53)	54
45	ANGLE OF MANDIBLE	ANGLE OF MANDIBLE	B				Gingivitis, rhinitis, pharyngitis, periodontal disease, halitosis	55
46	MANDIBULAR RAMUS	MANDIBULAR RAMUS	B				Pimples, acne	56
47	TONSIL	TONSIL	V				Lesions on face and mouth, white patches on mucous membrane	56
48	CHIN	CHIN	V				Herpes, fever, dryness in face, dry cracked lips	57
49	INFRA-MENTAL TUBERCLE	INFRA-MENTAL TUBERCLE	B				Oral problems	57
50	INFRA-MENTAL TUBERCLE	GONION (L)	B				Halitosis, rheumatoid arthritis	58
51	SUBMANDIBULAR	SUBMANDIBULAR	B				Oral dental, cavity problems, sinus abscess, breast masses	58
52	CORPUS CALLOSUM	CORPUS CALLOSUM	S				Addiction to drugs or alcohol, epilepsy, dyslexia	59
53	CORPUS CALLOSUM (Center)	CORPUS CALLOSUM (L Border)	B				TB, brain fog, headaches, bacterial meningitis	59
54	PINEAL	PINEAL	V, B				Psycho/emotional issues, insomnia, anxiety	60
55	PINEAL	CEREBELLUM	S				Hair loss	60
56	PINEAL	MEDULLA	V				Guillain Barre, shortness of breath, numbness in finger tips	61
57	PINEAL	BREAST	S				Can improve lactation	61
58	POST PINEAL	BLADDER	F				Neurological and behavioral disorders, fatigue, fevers, cough	62
59	PARIETAL	PARIETAL	V				Brain fog or inflammation, excessive secretion mucous membrane	62
60	PARIETAL (L or R)	TRANSVERSE COLON	P				Headaches, neck tension, vomiting, seizures, contaminated food	63
61	PARIETAL	KIDNEY (Contralateral)	S				Goiz Pair, Leg length discrepancy, Emotional strength	63
62	TEMPORAL	TEMPORAL	B				Rickettsia, Lyme, insomnia, headaches, muscle aches	64
63	TEMPORAL (R)	TEMPORAL (R)	S, E				Extreme aggressiveness, loss of humor, cold feet	64
64	TEMPORAL (L)	TEMPORAL (L)	V				Anorexia, mood swings, insomnia, respiratory symptoms	65
65	TEMPORAL	MEDULLA	V				Coronavirus	65
66	EXTERNAL EAR	EXTERNAL EAR	S				Intoxications, nervous ticks, facial paralysis, drooping eyelid	66

Dr. GARCIA
BIOMAGNETISM
Therapy • Training • Products

Dr. Garcia's Biomagnetism Scan Sheet

R = Reservoir, B = Bacteria, V = Virus, P = Parasite, F = Fungus, S = Special, D = Dysfunction, T = Trauma, E = Emotional

				S # 1	S # 2	S # 3	INTERPRETATION	PAGE
67	INNER EAR	INNER EAR	P				Toxoplasmosis; tinnitus; affects cats, birds, and dogs	66
68	TEMPOROOCCIPITAL	TEMPOROOCCIPITAL	B				Pneumonia, brain fog	67
69	OCCIPITAL	OCCIPITAL	V, E				EBV, fatigue, schizophrenia, bipolar, depression, sleep issues	68
70	CEREBELLUM	CEREBELLUM	S				Epilepsy, panic attacks, lockjaw, teeth grinding	68
71	MEDULLA	CEREBELLUM	V				Raw poultry, vertigo, sleep apnea, conjunctivitis, flu symptoms	69
72	MEDULLA	THYROID	V				Headaches, shortness of breath	69
73	MEDULLA	HEART	S, E				Bradycardia, helps regulate normal heart rhythm	70
74	MEDULLA	BLADDER	V				Fever, shortness of breath, vomiting, headaches, muscle/joint pain	70
NECK								
75	LARYNX	LARYNX	B				Pertussis, hyperthyroidism, violent coughing	71
76	THYROID	THYROID	D				Hyper-, hypothyroidism, uppershoulder infections	71
77	PARATHYROID	PARATHYROID	D				Physical and psychic stimulants, gastrointestinal/thryroid issues	72
78	CAROTID ARTERY	CAROTID ARTERY	S				High blood pressure, strokes, arterial hypertension	72
79	SCM (Sternocleidomastoid)	SCM (Sternocleidomastoid)	D				Low BP, bad circulation, perspiration, palpitations, irritable colon	73
80	VAGUS NERVE	KIDNEY (Contralateral)	R				Universal Reservoir, frequently bacterial	73
81	CERVICAL PLEXUS	CERVICAL PLEXUS	S, B				Food poisoning, halitosis, bladder/prostate infections, low energy	74
82	C1 VERTEBRA	C1 VERTEBRA	S				Lack or excess of sexual desire, mood swings	75
83	C1 VERTEBRA	PYLORUS	P				Malaria fibromyalgia	75
84	C3 VERTEBRA	BLADDER	P				Malaria, fibromyalgia, neck pain or stiffness	76
85	C3 VERTEBRA	SUPRASPINATUS	P				Seizures, insufficient respiration, liquid retention	76
86	C7 VERTEBRA	C7 VERTEBRA	P				Epilepsy, whiplash, numbness or weakness in the arm	77
87	C7 VERTEBRA	T1 VERTEBRA	S				Acute pain in neck and elbow	77
88	C7 VERTEBRA	SACRUM	D				Sweaty palms, poor circulation, palpitations, IBS, heaadaches	78

Dr. Garcia's Biomagnetism Scan Sheet

R = Reservoir, B = Bacteria, V = Virus, P = Parasite, F = Fungus, S = Special, D = Dysfunction, T = Trauma, E = Emotional

				S # 1	S # 2	S # 3	INTERPRETATION	PAGE
THORAX								
89	SUPRASPINATUS	SUPRASPINATUS	B				TB, shortness of breath, gall or kidney stones, calcium buildup	81
90	SUBCLAVIAN	SUBCLAVIAN	B				Pulmonary symptoms, swelling, edemas, non Hodgkin's lymphoma	82
91	MANUBRIUM	MANUBRIUM	V				Problems with larynx, nose, and airways, meningitis, pericarditis	82
92	1st RIB	1st RIB	F				Tinea capitis (scalp), athlete's foot, jock itch, ringworm	83
93	PECTORALIS MAJOR	PECTORALIS MAJOR	B				Respiratory problems, transmitted by bird feathers	83
94	CORONARY	LUNG (L)	B				Coronary obstructions, heart attacks	84
95	AORTIC KNOB	T7 VERTEBRA	B				Asphyxia, respiratory problems	84
96	PERICARDIUM	PERICARDIUM	B				Pericarditis, endocarditis, arrhythmia, cardiac pathologies	85
97	HEART	FALSE RIB (L)	S		﹀		Chronic bronchitis, emphysema, respiratory disorders	85
98	ATRIOVENTRICULAR NODE	KIDNEY (L)	S, V				Tachycardia, arrhythmia, German measles, heart palpitations	86
99	MEDIASTINUM	MEDIASTINUM	B				Immunodeficiency commonly misdiagnosed as AIDS	87
100	THYMUS	THYMUS	D				Thymus dysfunction, Key to Vital Energy	87
101	THYMUS	PARIETAL (R or L)	V				German measles	88
102	THYMUS	SPLEEN	S				Shortness of breath, smokers	88
103	THYMUS	ADRENAL	S				Hormonal equilibrium, menopause, oral ulcers	89
104	THYMUS	RECTUM	V				HIV, E. coli	89
105	THYMUS	PENIS or CLITORIS	S				Erectile dysfunction	90
106	CARINA	CARINA	V				Coughing, bronchitis, cold sores in mouth, transmitted by dairy	90
107	TRACHEA	TRACHEA	V				Common cold, laryngitis, sinusitis, otitis	91
108	STERNUM	ADRENAL	S				Spleen malfunctions, hematic disorders, chronic anemia	91
109	ESOPHAGUS	ESOPHAGUS	P				Anorexia, jaundice, digestive, tracheal, and cardiac problems	92
110	ESOPHAGUS	BLADDER	F				Exposure to bat excrement, insufficient respiration, SOB	92
111	PLEURAL	PLEURAL	V				Painful dry cough on both sides of ribs	93
112	PLEURAL (L)	PLEURAL (L)	B				Coughing with a lot of phlegm, asphyxia	93

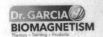

Dr. Garcia's Biomagnetism Scan Sheet

R = Reservoir, B = Bacteria, V = Virus, P = Parasite, F = Fungus, S = Special, D = Dysfunction, T = Trauma, E = Emotional

				S # 1	S # 2	S # 3	INTERPRETATION	PAGE
113	PLEURAL (R)	LIVER	V				Fatigue, malaise, appetite lose, jaundice, dark urine, abdomin pain	94
114	LUNG	LUNG	B				Tuberculosis, shortness of breath, gall or kidney stones	94
115	COSTAL CARTILAGE 6	COSTAL CARTILAGE 6	F				Chronic cough, bronchitis	95
116	FRONT	ADRENAL	S				Asthma	95
ABDOMEN								
117	CARDIAC SPHINCTER	PYLORUS	B				Gastric and digestive issues, reflux	97
118	CARDIAC SPHINCTER	APPENDIX	B				Bartonella, Lyme, severe digestive problems	97
119	CARDIAC SPHINCTER	ADRENAL	B				Gluten intolerance, reumatic fever, joint pain, reflux	98
120	ESOPHAGEAL HIATUS	ESOPHAGEAL HIATUS	P				Nausea, vomiting, hiccups, abdominal pain, bloating, diarrhea	98
121	ESOPHAGEAL HIATUS	ESOPHAGUS	B				Pulmonary problems, pneumonitis, accentuated halitosis, hernias	99
122	ESOPHAGEAL HIATUS	TESTICLE or VAGINA (R)	B				Pyloric and duodenal ulcers, gastritis, hiatal hernias, reflux	99
123	UPPER LIVER	UPPER LIVER	B				Asthma, emphysema, insufficient respiration, abdominal pain	100
124	STOMACH	STOMACH	D				Stomach cramps, indigestion, belching, gastritis, halitosis, acidity	100
125	STOMACH	THYMUS	B				Red sandy eyes, fatigue, disheveled face	101
126	STOMACH	PYLORUS	B				Gastritis, digestive disorders, diabetes, stomach cancer	101
127	STOMACH	LIVER	S				Unsatiatiated appetite	102
128	STOMACH	TRANSVERSE COLON	B				Fever, chills, headache, malaise, myalgia, respiratory tract	102
129	STOMACH	ADRENAL	V				Measles, MMR vaccine	103
130	STOMACH	SACRUM	B				Intestinal pain and bleeding, hiatal hernia	103
131	PANCREATIC BELT		S				Diebetes (Also p. 169)	104
132	PANCREAS HEAD	PYLORUS	B				Colitis, IBS, Chrohn's, metastasis, diabetes, diarrhea	104
133	PANCREAS HEAD	ADRENAL	B				Diabetes, gastroesophageal reflux, gluten intolerance	105
134	PANCREAS BODY	STOMACH	S				Food allergies (when not justified w/ other pair)	105
135	PANCREAS BODY	PANCREAS TAIL	S, V				Improves digestion, obesity, drug intoxication (Also p. 104)	106

Dr. Garcia's Biomagnetism Scan Sheet

R = Reservoir, B = Bacteria, V = Virus, P = Parasite, F = Fungus, S = Special, D = Dysfunction, T = Trauma, E = Emotional

				S#1	S#2	S#3	INTERPRETATION	PAGE
136	PANCREAS BODY	SPLEEN	P				Flatworms (from horses and pets)	107
137	PANCREAS TAIL	SPLEEN	V				Common warts (HPV)	107
138	PANCREAS TAIL	LIVER	B				Abdominal paine, shortness breath, nausea	108
139	PANCREAS TAIL	DUODENUM	P/V				Raw fish, intestinal discomfort, diabetes, obesity	108
140	PANCREAS TAIL	KIDNEY (L)	S				Arsenic Poisoning, fatigue	109
141	SPLEEN	SPLEEN	D, B				Blood disorders, leprosy, TB (Also p. 77)	109
142	SPLEEN	LUNG (L)	R				Immune system, respiratory issues	110
143	SPLEEN	LIVER	B				Pulmonary and liver symptomatology, blood disorders	111
144	PANCREATIC LIGAMENT	SPLEEN	V				High fever, headache, vomitting, muscle and joint pain	111
145	PANCREATIC LIGAMENT	DESCENDING COLON	V				Yellow Fever Virus, jaundice, hemorrhages	112
146	PERI-PANCREATIC	PERI-PANCREATIC	V				Laryngeal problems, otitis, chronic sinusitis, asthma, rage	112
147	PANCREATIC DUCT	KIDNEY (L)	B				Diabetes, food intolerances, indigestion	113
148	PYLORUS	PYLORUS	D				Abnormal contraction of pylorus	113
149	PYLORUS	TONGUE	P				Trichinosis, muscular and joint pain, vomiting, diarrhea, anorexia	114
150	PYLORUS	LIVER	P				Pinworms, malnutrition, gastrinal pain, anal itching, empty feeling	114
151	PYLORUS	TRANSVERSE COLON	S				Unsatiatiated appetite from anxiety, swallowing instead of eating	115
152	PYLORUS	URETER (L)	F				Diarrhea, expulsion of mucous ball, bad digestion, abdominal pain	115
153	PYLORUS	KIDNEY (L)	P				Vomit or metal taste in mouth, malabsorption of food, abscesses	116
154	LIVER	LIVER	T				High cholesterol, jaundice, pain, digestive disorders, fatigue	116
155	LIVER	PYLORUS	B				Hepatic abscess, cirrhosis (found in dairy, deli meats, and hot dogs)	117
156	LIVER	KIDNEY (L)	P				Hepatic abscess, false diabetes, false metastasis to the liver	117
157	LIVER	KIDNEY (R)	S				Hepatic cirrhosis, fatty liver	118
158	HEPATIC LIGAMENT	KIDNEY (R)	V				Roseola, fever, abdominal bloating, inflammation of glands	118
159	LIVER (Posterior)	KIDNEY (R)	S				Fatigue, irritability, low spirit, metal poisoning	119

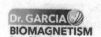

Dr. Garcia's Biomagnetism Scan Sheet

R = Reservoir, B = Bacteria, V = Virus, P = Parasite, F = Fungus, S = Special, D = Dysfunction, T = Trauma, E = Emotional

			S #1	S #2	S #3	INTERPRETATION	PAGE
160	LIVER (Posterior)	KIDNEY (R)	P				Psoriasis, baldness, hepatic scabies	119
161	DIAPHRAGM	DIAPHRAGM	F				Fungus infecting skin, genitals, throat, mouth, and blood	120
162	DIAPHRAGM (R or L)	KIDNEY (Homolateral)	B				Causes miscarriages and premature birth	120
163	COSTODIAPHRAGMATIC (L)	COSTODIAPHRAGMATIC (L)	P				Pancreatitis, anemia, leukemia, cardiac insufficiency, diabetes	121
164	LIVER COSTAL MARGIN (R)	LIVER	B				Borrelia burgdorferi, Lyme, simulates cirrhosis or hep C	121
165	COSTAL	COSTAL	B				Sharp chest pain with breathing	122
166	ANTERIOR COSTAL	ANTERIOR COSTAL	V				Ebola	122
167	GALLBLADDER	KIDNEY (R)	V				Common cold, sudden intense sneezing, watery nasal discharge	123
168	SUBDIAPHRAGM	SUBDIAPHRAGM	R				Abdominal distention	123.
169	PORTAL VEIN	PORTAL VEIN	B				Pneumonia	124
170	BELOW LIVER	BELOW LIVER	B				Loss of strength and energy, diarrhea, fever, enlarged liver	124
171	GALL BLADDER DUCT	KIDNEY (R or L)	B				False diabetes, indigestion, abdominal bloating	5.25
172	JEJUNUM	JEJUNUM	D, R				Universal Reservoir, IBS, abdominal pain, flatulence, bloating	125
173	ILEUM	ILEUM	S				Constipation, intestinal sluggishness	126
174	BELLY BUTTON	BELLY BUTTON	S				Thrombosis	126
175	OMENTUM	OMENTUM	B				Acne and other skin problems	127
176	DUODENUM	DUODENUM	D				Irritable colon, nervous colitis	127
177	DUODENUM	SPLEEN	R				Leukemia, pulmonary problems, anemia, Yersinia	128
178	DUODENUM	LIVER	B				Hep D, urogenital infectinos, infertility in women	128
179	DUODENUM	KIDNEY (L)	B				Vaginal/rectal bleeding, diabetes, infertility, low platelet count	129
180	ASCENDING COLON	ASCENDING COLON	B				Digestive problems, meningitis, endocarditis, pneumonia	129
181	ASCENDING COLON	DESCENDING COLON	V				Herpes, ulcerations and scabs in affected area	130
182	ASCENDING COLON	LIVER	B				Hep E, colitis, bad digestion, bleeding, lung problems	130
183	ASCENDING COLON	KIDNEY (R)	B				Pneumonia, urinary tract, soft tissue infections, surgical wound	131

Dr. Garcia's Biomagnetism Scan Sheet

R = Reservoir, B = Bacteria, V = Virus, P = Parasite, F = Fungus, S = Special, D = Dysfunction, T = Trauma, E = Emotional

				S # 1	S # 2	S # 3	INTERPRETATION	PAGE
184	ASCENDING COLON	SACRUM	B				Cystic fibrosis, pneumonia, lung problems	131
185	TRANSVERSE COLON	TRANSVERSE COLON	D				IBS, colitis, irritable colon, abdominal spasms, constipation	132
186	TRANSVERSE COLON	LIVER	B				Cholera, hepatitis symptoms	132
187	TRANSVERSE COLON	BLADDER	B				Diarrhea, flatulence, abdominal swelling, diabetes	133
188	DESCENDING COLON	DESCENDING COLON	B				Colitis, irritable colon, gas, distention of colon, rectal bleeding	133
189	DESCENDING COLON	LIVER	B, V				Hep A, jaundice, fatigue, lack of appetite, muscle pain	134
190	DESCENDING COLON	KIDNEY (L)	B				Distension, colic pain gases, vaginal bleeding, urinary infections	134
191	DESCENDING COLON	RECTUM	S				Acute pain and inflammation in digestive tract	135
192	DESCENDING COLON	QUADRICEPS (L)	P				Flatworm, skin hypersensitivity, dermatitis, pain in iliac fossa	135
193	CECUM	CECUM	P				Vaginal infections with bad smell and leucorrhoea	136
194	ILEOCECAL VALVE	KIDNEY (L)	P				Vaginal infections, vaginal discharge and painful urination	136
195	APPENDIX	TONGUE (L)	V				Smallpox, flat warts, dermatitis, acne, vaginitis	137
196	APPENDIX	THYMUS	S				Immunodeficiencies (leukemia, cancer, HIV, etc.)	137
197	APPENDIX	PLEURA	B				Appendicitis; laryngeal, trachea, pleura, and eye problems	138
198	APPENDIX	FEMORAL VEIN (Anterior) (L)	V				Smallpox vaccination, prostate issues, widespread rash	138
199	CONTRACECUM	CONTRACECUM	B				Flatulence, rectal, vaginal discharge, diarrhea, varicose veins	139
200	URETER	URETER	V				Chicken Pox, urinary tract infection, female infertility	139
201	SIGMOID	RECTUM	V				Nutrient deficiencies, demineralization, low energy in children	140
POSTERIOR THORAX								
202	VENA CAVA	VENA CAVA	F				Athlete's foot, ringworm, vaginal itching, hair loss	143
293	LATISSIMUS	LATISSIMUS	B				Pneumonia, halitosis, fluid build up in lungs, heart issues	143
204	T2 VERTEBRA	T2 VERTEBRA	B				Legionnaire's disease, upper and lower airway symptoms	144
205	T3 VERTEBRA	T3 VERTEBRA	B				Avian TB,	144
206	T3 VERTEBRA	T7 VERTEBRA	V				Foot and mouth, dairy, ulcers, upper back pain	145
207	T5 VERTEBRA	L4 VERTEBRA	B				Spina bifida, inflammation of the meninges and nerves, arthritis	145

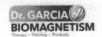

Dr. Garcia's Biomagnetism Scan Sheet

R = Reservoir, B = Bacteria, V = Virus, P = Parasite, F = Fungus, S = Special, D = Dysfunction, T = Trauma, E = Emotional

			S #1	S #2	S #3	INTERPRETATION	PAGE
208	ADRENAL	ADRENAL	D				Chronic fatigue, low blood pressure, tetanus, TB, strep	146
209	RENAL CAPSULE	RENAL CAPSULE	B				Lupus, butterfly pigmentation	147
210	KIDNEY	KIDNEY	D, B				Tetanus, muscular pains, lumbar pain, mental confusion (Also 182)	147
211	KIDNEY (L)	URETER (L)	S				Kidney stones, menstrual symptoms, ureter pain	148
212	RENAL CALYX	URETER	V				Herpes, false diabetes, PMS	149
213	PARAVERTEBRAL	PARAVERTEBRAL	S				Back pain	149
214	PERIRENAL	PERIRENAL	B				Raw milk, TB, boils, pimples, foruncles, carbuncles	150
215	FLOATING RIB	FLOATING RIB	B				Yersinia, digestive tract,	151
216	QUADRATUS LUMBORUM	QUADRATUS LUMBORUM	B				Syphilis, ulcers in mouth, back pain, degenerative hips	151
217	L4 VERTEBRA	L4 VERTEBRA	B				Gonorrhea, halitosis, lumbar pain, urogenitaal symptoms, arthritis	152
218	L5 VERTEBRA	L5 VERTEBRA	B				Lower back pain, weakness, numbness, shooting pain down leg	153
219	ILIUM	ILIUM	S				Constipation, abdominal discomfort, weight issues, varicose veins	153
220	ILIAC CREST	ILIAC CREST	P				Sleeping sickness, digestive disorders, extreme fatigue	154
221	LUMBAR PLEXUS	LUMBAR PLEXUS	B				Diarrhea, rectal bleeding, digestive tract problems	154
222	DOUGLAS SACK (L)	FEMORAL VEIN (Anterior) (L)	V				Vomitting together with diarrhea, food poisoning	155
223	CAUDA EQUINA	CAUDA EQUINA	V				Burning/stinging pain and numbness in leg, cold sores	155
224	SACRUM	SACRUM	B				Low back pain, nerve discomfort in lower limbs, infertility	156
225	SACRUM	KIDNEY (L)	D				Intestinal noises, flatulence, intestinal laziness (Also 182)	156
226	RECTUM	RECTUM	B				Cancer metastasis	157
227	RECTUM	ANUS	S				Diarrhea, rectal discomfort or pain	157
228	RECTUM	THYMUS	V				HIV	158
ARMS								
229	AXILLA	AXILLA	V				Digestive problems, ear issues, asthma, back pain, insomnia	161
230	AXILLA (Retro)	AXILLA (Retro)	B				Problems with shoulder girdle, lungs, digestive system, mouth	161
231	NEUROVASCULAR BUNDL-ARM	NEUROVASCULAR BUNDLE-ARM	F				Throat and neck, bad underarm odor, bursitis	162

Dr. Garcia's Biomagnetism Scan Sheet

R = Reservoir, B = Bacteria, V = Virus, P = Parasite, F = Fungus, S = Special, D = Dysfunction, T = Trauma, E = Emotional

				S # 1	S # 2	S # 3	INTERPRETATION	PAGE
232	NEUROVASCULAR BUNDL-ARM	ELBOW	B				Strep, throat and/or skin issues	162
233	DELTOID INSERTION	DELTOID INSERTION	B				Carpal Tunnel, frozen shoulder (turn body to look behind)	163
234	DELTOID	DELTOID	B				Oral and joint problems, peridontal disease, thyroid	163
235	DELTOID	KIDNEY (L)	P				Skin ulcers, fever, low RBC, enlarged spleen and liver	164
236	HUMERUS	HUMERUS	B				Pneumonia, transmitted by dogs	164
237	BRACHIAL	BRACHIAL	B				Strep, psoriasis–like	165
238	ELBOW	ELBOW	S				Fungal infections, white dry scaly elbow, eye issues	165
239	ULNA	ULNA	V				Herpes, burning sensation on face, esp. lips, or other body part	166
240	RADIUS	RADIUS	F				Herpes, ringworm and other skin problems incl. dandruff	166
241	WRIST	WRIST	B				Rickettsia, Alzheimer's	167
242	PALM	PALM	P				Malaria, fibromyalgia, sweaty or cold clammy hands/feet	167
243	INDEX	INDEX	B				E coli, urinary tract infections, rectal bleeding	168
PELVIS								
244	SUPRAPUBIC	SUPRAPUBIC	V				Jock itch, male infertility	171
245	UTERUS	UTERUS	S, R				Digestive symptoms, vomiting, bulimia (Also p. 161)	171
246	UTERUS	OVARY	D, R				Pregnancy identification (can be false) (Also p. 162)	172
247	UTERUS	SACRUM	S				Endometriosis, uterine hemorrhage	172
248	FALLOPIAN TUBE	FALLOPIAN TUBE	V				Infertility, (dogs, cats), vaginal bleeding	173
249	FALLOPIAN TUBE	OVARY (Homolateral)	S				Helps avoid ectopic pregnancies (Also p. 162)	173
250	OVARY/TESTICLE	OVARY or TESTICLE	D				Balances menses, early menopause, excess hair on women (168)	174
251	BLADDER	BLADDER	D, B				Urinary tract infection, incontinence, kidney stones, psoriasis	174
252	BLADDER	BLADDER	V				Genital herpes, burning rash in genital region and/or legs, NS	175
253	BLADDER	ANUS	S				Pelvic bleeding, pelvic issues	176
254	BLADDER	RECTUM	B				Diarrhea, hemorrhoids, flatulance	176
255	INGUINAL NERVE	VAGINA	V				Dryness in crotch, low back pain, leukemia/lymph	177

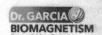

Dr. Garcia's Biomagnetism Scan Sheet

R = Reservoir, B = Bacteria, V = Virus, P = Parasite, F = Fungus, S = Special, D = Dysfunction, T = Trauma, E = Emotional

#				S#1	S#2	S#3	INTERPRETATION	PAGE
256	INGUINAL NERVE (L)	INGUINAL NERVE	V				Roseola, Joint pain, roseola	177
257	ADNEXA	LIVER	V				Infertility, vaginal or anal discomfort, protruding bulges in vagina	178
258	PUDENDAL NERVE	ADNEXA	V				Mumps, inflammation on one side of neck, male infertility	178
259	SPHINCTER OF URETHRA	PUDENDAL NERVE	V				Incontinence, burning sensation while urinating	179
260	URETHRA	SPHINCTER OF URETHRA	V				Frequent urination, rectal bleeding, cystitis, cervical dysplasia, RSV	179
261	SPERMATIC CORD	URETHRA	B, R				Insomnia, chronic cough, inflammation of the kidney, infertility	180
262	VAS DEFERENS	SPERMATIC CORD	V				Recurrent fevers, laryngeal problems and dry coughs	180
263	VAGINA	LARYNX	B				Yersinia pestis, vaginal discharge, dry cough	181
264	TESTICLE	VAGINA (Horizontal)	B				Vaginal discharge, dry cough, anemia, leukemia	181
265	CLITORIS	TESTICLE	B				Vaginal/rectal irritation with bleeding, pelvic inflammation	182
266	CLITORIS	CLITORIS	B				Lyme's Disease	182
267	PROSTATE	SACRUM	D				Prostate dysfunction, flatulence, gaseous, intestinal laziness	183
268	PROSTATE	PROSTATE	V				HPV, anal lesions	183
LEGS								
269	GLUTEUS	GLUTEUS	P				Large intestinal parasites	185
270	GLUTEUS (L)	PYLORUS	B				Digestive issues, paracarditis	185
271	GLUTEUS (L)	FEMORAL VEIN (Posterior) (L)	P				Babesia, brain fog, tumoral growth	186
272	GREATER SCIATIC NOTCH	GREATER SCIATIC NOTCH	B				Sinus, eye issues, headaches, diarrhea, sciatica, scoliosis	186
273	ISCHIAL RAMUS	ISCHIAL RAMUS	B				Flatulence and constipation, mucous secretions	187
274	COCCYX	COCCYX	V				Rotavirus, uncomfortable when sitting, diarrhea	187
275	ANUS	ANUS	V				Warts, hemorrhoids, myomas	188
276	ANUS	PYLORUS	F				Vaginal yeast infection, digestive issues	188
277	ISCHIUM	ISCHIUM	P				Digestive issues, bloated stomach, anal itching, rectal bleeding	189
278	SCIATIC	SCIATIC	V				Scoliosis, paralysis or weakness in lower back	189
279	FEMORAL FOSSA	FEMORAL FOSSA	V				Herpes, jock itch, roseola, dermatitis	190

Dr. Garcia's Biomagnetism Scan Sheet

R = Reservoir, B = Bacteria, V = Virus, P = Parasite, F = Fungus, S = Special, D = Dysfunction, T = Trauma, E = Emotional

			S # 1	S # 2	S # 3	INTERPRETATION	PAGE
280	POPLITEAL FOSSA	POPLITEAL FOSSA	B				Pneumonia, coughing upon exposure to cold air,	190
281	POPLITEAL FOSSA (L)	INGUINAL NERVE (L)	V				Herpes, jock itch	191
282	ACHILLES	ACHILLES	B				Digestive issues, pain in legs, headache, fever, malaise	191
283	CALCANEUS	CALCANEUS	B				Contributes to Alzheimer's	192
284	GREATER TROCHANTER	GREATER TROCHANTER	B				Diarrhea, lower back pain, diabetes, typhoid fever	192
285	GREATER TROCHANTER	KIDNEY (L)	B				Salmonella, diarrhea, weakness, stomach pain, headache	193
286	GREATER TROCHANTER (L)	TENSOR FASCIAE LATAE	F				Fever, chills, skin lesions	193
287	LESSER TROCHANTER	LESSER TROCHANTER	V				Vaginitis, yeast infections, discomfort in the crotch	194
288	ADDUCTOR	ADDUCTOR	V				HIV, itching, burning in pubic area, vaginal/rectal bleeding	194
289	TENSOR FASCIAE LATAE	TENSOR FASCIAE LATAE	B				Itching, burning	195
290	TENSOR FASCIAE LATAE (Retro)	PECTORALIS MAJOR (L)	V				Warts, skin tags	195
291	QUADRICEPS	QUADRICEPS	S				Pain in lower limbs, waist, hip, pelvis; detox from pesticides	196
292	PATELLA	PATELLA	B				Fear, anxiety, depression, bipolar, arrythmias, MS	196
293	EXTERNAL KNEE LIGAMENT (L)	QUADRATUS LUMBORUM (L)	B				Miscarriage, pelvic inflammation, endometriosis, dermatitis	197
294	MEDIAL KNEE LIGAMENT (L)	MEDIAL MALLEOLUS (L)	F				Hair and skin infections, dandruff, knee and ankle pain, Ringworm	197
295	PES ANSERINE	PES ANSERINE	V				COVID 19, knee pain	198
296	TIBIA	TIBIA	V					198
PERSONAL PAIRS							
297	MOLE	KIDNEY (Homolateral)	V				Common cold symptoms with fatigue, headache, cough	215
298	BLADDER	TRAUMA	T				Trauma pain	216
299	TRAUMA	KIDNEY	T				Trauma pain	216
300	INGUINAL NERVE	PAIN	T				Joint pain, inflammation, infection, drainage	217
301	DOG BITE	ARMPIT	R				Reservoir for rabies	219

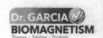

Dr. Garcia's Biomagnetism Scan Sheet

R = Reservoir, B = Bacteria, V = Virus, P = Parasite, F = Fungus, S = Special, D = Dysfunction, T = Trauma, E = Emotional

				S#1	S#2	S#3	INTERPRETATION	PAGE
EMOTIONAL PAIRS								
302	HIPPOCAMPUS	AMYGDALA	E				Loneliness	221
303	AMYGDALA	THYMUS	E				Hate	221
304	CENTRAL SULCUS	CENTRAL SULCUS	E				Feeling superior	222
305	PINEAL	PROSTATE or UTERUS	E				Lust, messy uncontrollable sexual desires	222
306	POST PINEAL	POST PINEAL	E				People who lie, invent, or deceive, often very intelligent	223
307	POST PINEAL	AMYGDALA	E				Depression	223
308	SYLVIAN FISSURE	SYLVIAN FISSURE	E				May increase creativity	224
309	OCCIPITAL	TESTICLE	E				Evil desires	224
310	MEDULLA	HEART	E				Cruelty (Also p. 228)	225
311	C1 VERTEBRA	UTERUS	E				Jealosy	225
312	HEART	PANCREAS	E				Envy	226
313	THYMUS	PITUITARY	E				Eagerness or excessive desire to have wealth	226
314	THYMUS	OVARY or TESTICLE	E				Impatience, don't like to wait, always in a hurry	227
315	TRACHEA	HEART	E				Intolerance	227
316	LUNG	LUNG	E				Guilt	228
317	LUNG (L)	MEDULLA	E				Sadness (when grieving)	228
318	STOMACH	HEART	E				Gluttony, obesity, desire pleasure with food	229
319	SPLEEN	HYPOTHALAMUS	E				Laziness	229
320	LIVER	HEART	E				Anger, feeling rights violated	230
321	TRANSVERSE COLON	OVARY or TESTICLE	E				Materialism	230
322	BELLY BUTTON	TESTICLE	E				Dependency on mother	231
323	BELLY BUTTON	UTERUS	E				Dependency on father, extreme rivalry to mother	231
324	ADRENAL	LIVER	E				Pride	232
325	BACK OF HAND	BACK OF HAND	E				Doubt	232

Dr. Garcia's Biomagnetism Scan Sheet

R = Reservoir, B = Bacteria, V = Virus, P = Parasite, F = Fungus, S = Special, D = Dysfunction, T = Trauma, E = Emotional

				S # 1	S # 2	S # 3	INTERPRETATION	PAGE
TUMORAL PHENOMENA								
326	Infiltrate	(V+V)	C					
327	Sjogren	(V + V + V)	C					
328	Exudate	(B or P or F) not a Virus	C					
329	Cyst or Polyp	(V+B)	C					
330	Abcess	(B+B) (90% False Cancer)	C					
331	Dysplasia	(B+B+V) Fast Growth!	C					
332	Benign Neoplasia Slow Growth (B+B+B+V)		C					
333	Benign Neoplasia Fast Growth (B+B+V+F) Explosive!		C					
334	Cancer (B+B+V+F+ Lepra) + Unresolved Emotion		C					
335	Metastasis (B+B+V+F+Pseodomona o Clostridium) + Lepra							
336	Septic Necrosis	(B+B+V+F+ Lepra+P)	C					
337	Association Zone	Kidney (right/Left) or Bladder	C					

NOTES

250

CANCER — The above "Tumor Phenomena" scan chart has the sequencing for the protocol to find location and whether it is a Virus (V), Bacteria (B), Parasite (P) or Fungus (F). For example, #330, Cyst or Polyop you would scan for Virus first, do placements, then find associated bacteria. Scan body to find where placements go. The chart below can be further used to locate cancerous growths. Per each tumor phenomena the placement protocols should be followed. V+V+V would mean you would search for a Virus and then another and then another if found #328 or "Sjogren" in the soul while scanning.

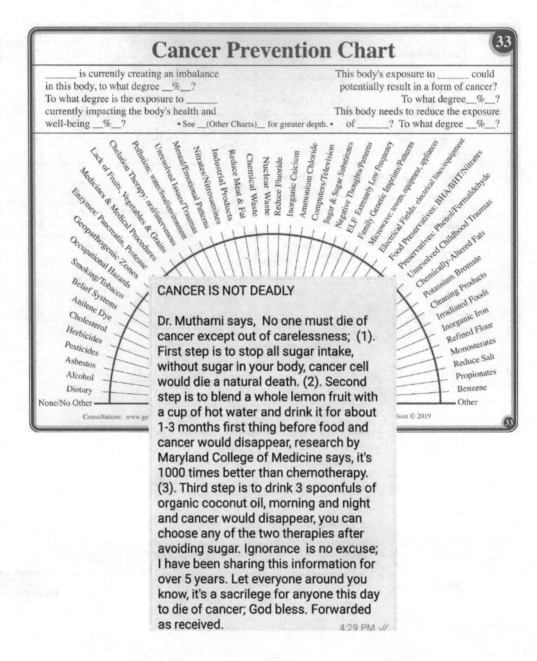

Cancer Prevention Chart ③③

_____ is currently creating an imbalance in this body, to what degree __%__? To what degree is the exposure to _____ currently impacting the body's health and well-being __%__?

This body's exposure to _____ could potentially result in a form of cancer? To what degree __%__? This body needs to reduce the exposure of _____? To what degree __%__?

• See __(Other Charts)__ for greater depth. •

Chelation Therapy: oral/intervenous
Lack of Fruits, Vegetables & Grains
Medicines & Medical Procedures
Enzymes: Pancreatin, Protease
Geopathogenic Zones
Occupational Hazards
Smoking/Tobacco
Belief Systems
Anilene Dye
Cholesterol
Herbicides
Pesticides
Asbestos
Alcohol
Dietary
None/No Other

Pollution: water/food/environment
Unresolved Issues/Traumas
Mental/Emotional Traumas
Nitrates/Nitrosamines
Industrial Products
Reduce Meat & Fat
Chemical Waste
Nuclear Waste
Reduce Fluoride
Inorganic Calcium
Ammonium Chloride
Computers/Television
Sugar & Sugar Substitutes
Negative Thoughts/Patterns
ELF Extremely Low Frequency
Family Genetic Imprints/Patterns
Microwave: towers, equipment, appliances
Electrical Fields: electrical lines/equipment
Food Preservatives: BHA/BHT/Nitrates
Preservatives: Phenol/Formaldehyde
Unresolved Childhood Traumas
Chemically-Altered Fats
Potassium Bromate
Cleaning Products
Irradiated Foods
Inorganic Iron
Refined Flour
Monosterates
Reduce Salt
Propionates
Benzene
Other

Consultations: www.ge...   ...lson © 2019

CANCER IS NOT DEADLY

Dr. Muthami says, No one must die of cancer except out of carelessness; (1). First step is to stop all sugar intake, without sugar in your body, cancer cell would die a natural death. (2). Second step is to blend a whole lemon fruit with a cup of hot water and drink it for about 1-3 months first thing before food and cancer would disappear, research by Maryland College of Medicine says, it's 1000 times better than chemotherapy. (3). Third step is to drink 3 spoonfuls of organic coconut oil, morning and night and cancer would disappear, you can choose any of the two therapies after avoiding sugar. Ignorance is no excuse; I have been sharing this information for over 5 years. Let everyone around you know, it's a sacrilege for anyone this day to die of cancer; God bless. Forwarded as received.   4:29 PM ✓✓

Covid Vaccine Placements

These placements are for Moderna and Pfizer vaccines. Try to get magnets placed withing 10 days of inoculation before it enters the entire system into the brain.

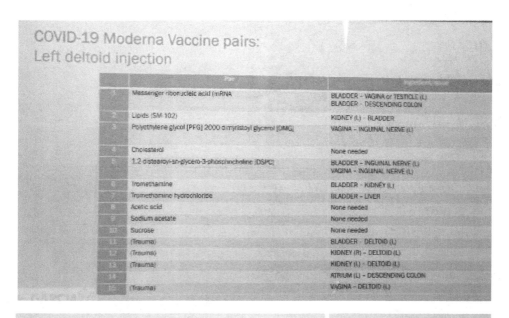

COVID-19 Moderna Vaccine pairs:
Left deltoid injection

#	Ingredient/issue	BioMagnetism Pair
1	Messenger ribonucleic acid (mRNA)	BLADDER – VAGINA or TESTICLE (L) BLADDER – DESCENDING COLON
2	Lipids (SM-102)	KIDNEY (L) – BLADDER
3	Polyethylene glycol [PEG] 2000 dimyristoyl glycerol [DMG]	VAGINA – INGUINAL NERVE (L)
4	Cholesterol	None needed
5	1,2 distearoyl-sn-glycero-3-phosphocholine [DSPC]	BLADDER – INGUINAL NERVE (L) VAGINA – INGUINAL NERVE (L)
6	Tromethamine	BLADDER – KIDNEY (L)
7	Tromethamine hydrochloride	BLADDER – LIVER
8	Acetic acid	None needed
9	Sodium acetate	None needed
10	Sucrose	None needed
11	(Trauma)	BLADDER – DELTOID (L)
12	(Trauma)	KIDNEY (R) – DELTOID (L)
13	(Trauma)	KIDNEY (L) – DELTOID (L)
14		ATRIUM (L) – DESCENDING COLON
15	(Trauma)	VAGINA – DELTOID (L)

D-19 Pfizer Vaccine pairs:
deltoid injection

#	Ingredient/issue	BioMagnetism Pair
1		DELTOID (R) – BLADDER
2		DELTOID (R) – KIDNEY (R)
3		DELTOID (R) – KIDNEY (L)
4		DELTOID (R) – TESTICLE (L)
5	mRNA Spike protein	BLADDER – TESTICLE (L)
6	mRNA Spike protein	BLADDER – TESTICLE (R)
7	1,2, distearoyl-sn-glycero-3-phosphocoline	BLADDER – BLADDER (Vertical)
8	1,2, distearoyl-sn-glycero-3-phosphocoline	FALLOPIAN TUBE (L) – TESTICLE (L)
9	Cholesterol	BLADDER – TESTICLE (L)
10	Cholesterol	ATRIUM (L) – LUNG (L)
11	(4-Hydroxybutyl) bis(hexane-6,1-diy	BLADDER – TESTICLE (L)
12	(4-Hydroxybutyl) bis(hexane-6,1-diy	BLADDER – TESTICLE (R)
13	Potassium Chloride	BLADDER – BLADDER (Vertical)
14	Monobasic Potassium Phosphate	INFERIOR MEDIASTINUM – BLADDER
15	More Drainage!!	BLADDER – TESTICLE (L)

These are ingredients of the JNJ and Astrozeneca vaxxines. You can muscle test with your soul to find what placements are needed. Remember to also scan the injection site for clearing as well. Additionally, below are listings of other vaccines issues to scan for.

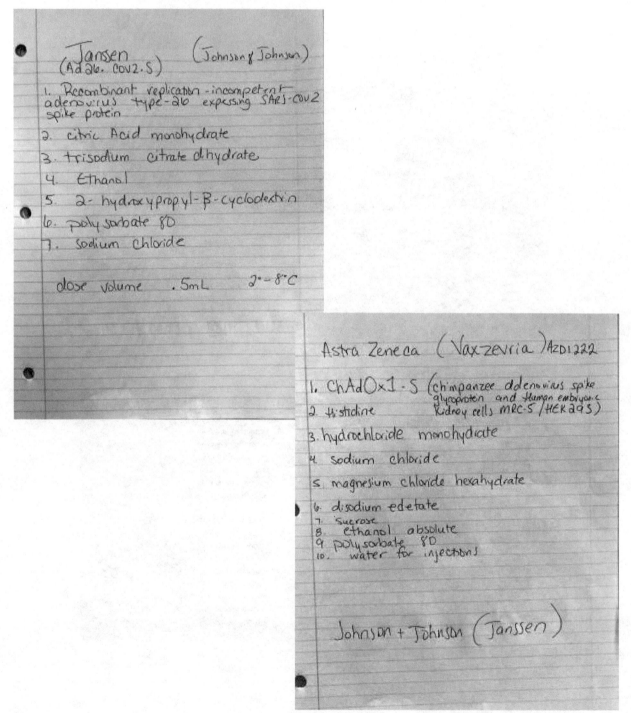

Janssen (Johnson y Johnson)
(Ad 26. COV2.S)

1. Recombinant replication-incompetent adenovirus type-26 expressing SARS-COV2 spike protein
2. citric Acid monohydrate
3. trisodium citrate dihydrate
4. Ethanol
5. 2-hydroxypropyl-β-cyclodextrin
6. polysorbate 80
7. Sodium chloride

dose volume .5mL   2°-8°C

Astra Zeneca (Vaxzevria) AZD1222

1. ChAdOx1-S (chimpanzee adenovirus spike glycoprotein and Human embryonic kidney cells MRC-5/HEK 293S)
2. histidine
3. hydrochloride monohydrate
4. sodium chloride
5. magnesium chloride hexahydrate
6. disodium edetate
7. sucrose
8. ethanol absolute
9. polysorbate 80
10. water for injections

Johnson + Johnson (Janssen)

Vaccine. Prion reservoir	36a	muscle control.
Vaccine. DPT	71a	Hyperthyroidism. Breathing
Vaccine. Mumps MMR	84a	Hormonal Production
Vaccine. Mumps MMR	52b	Nervous System. Testicular Inflamation
Vaccine.German Measles	88a	Damage to Eyes
Vaccine. German Measles	124b	Skin Rashes. Heart Palpatations. Eyes
Vaccine.English Measles	105a	Rash on Arms.Legs.Torso.GI bleeding.Fever.
Vaccine.Smallpox	161a	Warts.Blindness.acne.vaginitis.
Vaccine.Chicken Pox	164b	Infertility.Renal.Urinary.
Vaccine.Smallpox	137a	Prostate.Skin Problems
Vaccine. Mumps MMR	152b	Paratoid Glands.Infertility.Slow Sperm.
Vaccine.Polio	165b	Lack Vitality.Lack of Nutrient Absortion.
Vaccine.Mad Cow Disease		Prion Reserve
Vaccine	211b	Eye Clumsiness. Head.sjorens.cancer
Vaccine.English Measles MMR	202b	Sever Rash on Skin
Vaccine small pox	48b	Circle of Willis
Vaccine.Smallpox	206a	
Vaccine.HPV	183b	Prostate Disfunction
Vaccine.HPV	106b	Skin Infection. Mucous Membrane
Vaccine.HPV	107a	Fish eye on Sole of Foot
Vaccine Yellow Fever	108b **	Yellow Fever Jaundice

General Symptoms, Ailments and Issues

You can also scan and place by issues, ailments, symptoms and diseases. The 2nd column is the associated page # where the placement is referred to in Dr. Garcia's Biomag Practitioner's Guide 3.0.

Diseases	75b	Fibromyalgia
Malaria		
Malaria	167a	Fibromyalgia
Aids/HIV	89b	GI. Pulmonary. Immune Deficient
Aids/HIV	161a	Digestion.Ear.Asthma.back pain.thyroid.cancer
Aids/HIV	122b**	Immune Deficiency. Lymphatic
Aids/HIV	168a	Urinary, Odor. Thymus. E.coli
Aids/HIV	158a	GI. Descending Colon. Rectum
Aids/HIV	155b	Itching, Pubic. Restless Leg. Burning. Ms.sciatica.

Aids/HIV	89b	hep B. viral reservoir
Aids/HIV	152a	Kidney Disfunction
Lyme Disease	52a	Insomnia. Headaches. Nervous system. Fever
Lyme Disease	121b	Aches. Psychosis. Behavior. Liver. Digestive
Lyme Disease	95a**	Joint Pain. Fever. Diabetes. Strep throat
Lyme Disease	192a	Joint Pain. Muscle Weakness. Alzheimers
Lyme Disease	186a	Brain Toxins. False cancer
Herpes	52b	Commissure 2x
Herpes	57a	Mouth. Lip Mucous. Fever. Dryness. Zsarcoma.
Herpes	56b	lesions. reservior. pain
Herpes	117b	Hepatitis destruction.
Herpes	166a	Breast scabbing. Burning Skin. Midsection.
Herpes	149a	Urinary. Pelvis.
Herpes	190a	Sciatic leg. Itching Groin
Herpes	191a	Dryness in Crotch.
Herpes	137b	Warts. Blindness. acne. vaginitis.
Herpes	171a	Numbness in legs to lips. Burning.
Herpes	155b	Herpes. Leg numbness. Cold Sores.blister.pain
Cancer	52b	Mouth cancer
Cancer	101a	Diabetes. Digestive. Stomach. cancer
Cancer	104b	Diabetes. Pancreas
Cancer	121b	Lymphotic Organs
Cancer	140a	Nutrient deficiencies. SV 40 cancer.
Cancer	174a**	Kidney & Gall Stones. Skin Pigmentation.
Cancer	186a	Brain Toxins.
Polio	189b	Lack of Leg Strength.
Polio	PP	Occipital/Liver
Polio	PP	Chin/Descending Colon
Polio	163a	Quad 2X DDT
MS	57a	Eyes. Cataract. Liver. Retina Deformation.
MS	56a**	Brain Inflammation. Meningitis.
MS	74a	Sides of Neck. Bladder. Prostate. Nervous.
MS	88a**	Hepatatic Scabies. Psorasis. Baldness.
TB	81a	*Shortness Breath. Night Sweats. Hot Flashes*
TB	77a**	Enlarged Spleen.Yersina Species. Leukemia.
TB	78a**	Respiratory. Immune

TB	139a	Insomnia. Chronic Cough. Infertility.
TB	174a**	Kidney/Gall Stones.Skin Pigmentation.Eye.
TB	180b**	Fatty Tissue Kidneys. Pimples. Boils.
TB	59a	Shortness Breath. Night Sweats. Hot Flashes
TB	228a	Guilt.
TB	211a	Parasympathetic Dysfunction
Vaccine. Prion reservoir **Covid**	36a	muscle control. Covid
Vaccine. Mumps MMR Vaccine	84a	Hormonal Production. Mumps
MMR	52b	Nervous System. Testicular Inflammation
Vaccine.German Measles	88a	Damage to Eyes
Vaccine. German Measles	124b	Skin Rashes. Heart Palpitations. Eyes
Vaccine.English Measles	105a	Rash on Arms.Legs.Torso.GI Bleeding.Fever.
Vaccine.Smallpox	161a	Warts. Blindness. acne. vaginitis.
Vaccine.Chicken Pox	164b	Infertility. Renal. Urinary.
Vaccine.Smallpox	137a	Prostate. Skin Problems
Vaccine. Mumps MMR Vaccine	152b	Paratoid Glands. Infertility. Slow Sperm.
Vaccine.Polio	165b	Lack Vitality. Lack of Nutrient Absortion.
Vaccine	211b	Eye Clumsiness. Head. Sjorens cancer
Vaccine.English Measles MMR	202b	Sever Rash on Skin
Vaccine small pox	48b	Circle of Willis
Vaccine.Smallpox	206a	
Vaccine.HPV	183b	Prostate Disfunction
Vaccine.HPV	106b	Skin Infection. Mucous Membrane
Vaccine.HPV	107a	Fish eye on Sole of Foot
Vaccine Yellow Fever	108b **	Yellow Fever Jaundice
Common Cold	42b**	Frontal Sinusitis. Headache. Fever. Sore Throat
Common Cold	42b**	Mucus Membrane. Flu Symptoms.Eyes.Head.
Common Cold.flu	58a	Laryngitis. Sunusitis. Otitis.
Common Cold	52b	Facial Paralysis. Eye. Mouth. Sinus. Urinary
Common Cold	92b	Nasal. Sneezing.
Common Cold	172a	
Common Cold.Hanta	31a	Fatigue. headache. cough. fever
Common Cold	62a	Fatigue. headache. cough. fever. brain fog
Flu	42a	Headaches. Severe Mucous. Eye
	50a	Diarrhea.Headaches.GI.Vomitting.Abdomen. Eyes.
Flu		

Flu	97b	
Flu.Bird	216b	
Lymph Nodes	57b	Chiasm 2x
Non-Hodgkins Lymphoma	82a	Liquid Retention. Swelling.
Luekemia	76a**	Pulmonary. Liver. Spleen. Blood Dyscrasias
Luekemia	77a**	Blood. Throat. Genitals. Mouth.
Luekemia	77b**	Low White Blood Cells.
Yersinia Pestis	76b**	Spleen Disfunction. Cough. Vaginal Discharge
Diet	52a	Parotid 2X
Diet	87b**	Below Liver 2X
Diet.Obesity	92a	Hepatic Ligament -Kidney ®
Diet.Obesity	118b	Pancreas Body - Pancreas Tail
Diet.Food Allergy	105b	Pancreas Body - Stomach
Diet.Sushi.Obesity	107a	Pancreas Tail - Duodenum
Diet	134a	Descending Colon - Liver
Diet.Obesity	136b	Duodenum 2X
Diet	192a	Greater Trochanter 2X
Diet.Obesity	102a	Stomach - Liver
Diet.Obesity	115a	Pylorus-Transverse Colon
Diet.Obesity	114b	Pylorus-Liver
Addiction/Detox	53a	Bacteria. Viral
Addiction/Detox	66b	Nervous Tics. Facial Paralysis
Addiction/Detox	51a	Snorting Drugs. Nasal. Nose2x
Addiction/Detox	88b	Smokers. Shortness of Breath
Addiction/Detox	126b	Smoking. Birth control. Obesity
Addiction/Detox	105b	GI Discomfort
Addiction/Detox	106a	Pancreas Body -Pancreas Tail
Addiction/Detox	59a	Alcohol. Drugs.
Addiction/Detox	170b**	Alcohol. Buzz Kill. Kidney. Gout
Psychotic Drugs	40b	Pituitary 2x
Arthritis	205a**	
Arthritis	210b	Autoimmune Inflammation.
Asthma	138a	Digestion. Ear. Asthma. back pain.thyroid. rabies
Asthma	164b	Lung infections. Immune Suppressed
Asthma	95b	Allergy.

Diabetes	40b	Pituitary-Medula
Diabetes	74a**	Pacreatitis.leukemia.cardiac.GI
Diabetes	123a	Sphincter. Abdomen. Bloating. Digestion.
Diabetes	93b**	Food Allergy. Pancrease. Digestion
Diabetes	94a**	Joint Pain.Stomach.GI Gluten Intolerance.Ulcer.
Diabetes	103a	Skin Irritation. GI. Gluten Intolerance
Diabetes	103b	GI. Diarrhea. Pancreas
Diabetes	133a	Food Intolerance. Diarrhea.GI. Urinary.
Diabetes	117a**	Sex Diseases. Vagina.Eyes.Intestions.Bleeding.
Diabetes	149a	Urinary. Pelvis.
E Coli	89b	Immune Deficiency. Headache. Red Eye. Fatigue
Norwalk Virus	74b**	Lung. Respiratory. Chronic Cough.Bronchitis.
Ebola	122a	Fever. Headaches. Nose. Fatigue. Breathing.
Yersinia	77a**	Blood. Throat. Genitals. Mouth.Spleen.
Yersinia	77b**	Luekemia. Emotions. Pulmonary. Anemia.
Yersinia Pestis	181a	Vagina. Menopause. Hair. Cough.
Chicken Pox	139b	Urinary. Renal.
HTLV 1	177a	Low Back. Dryness. Urethra.
HTLV	194a	Vagina. Irritation. Genitals.
Yellow Fever	203a	Severe Rash Skin.
Leukemia	77b**	Pulmonary Amnesia
Leukema	137b	Immune Deficiency.
Pneumonia	83b	Children. Respiratory.
Pneumonia	124a	Liver. Lungs
Pneumonia	121a	Eye. Appendix. Immune Deficiency
Pneumonia	138b	Latissimus 2X
Pneumonia	190b	Popliteal 2X
Pneumonia	126b	Belly Button
Candida	120a	Bloodstream Infection. Immune.
Juandice	134a	Descending Colon - Liver
Juandice	92a	Esophagus 2X
Mononucleosis	68b	Occipital 2X
Lupus	212b	Renal Capsule 2X
Bronchitis	90b	Carina 2X
Bronchitis	131a	Ascending Colon - Kidney®

Bronchitis	165a	Brachial 2X
Bronchitis	157a**	Parietal - Kidney
Infertility	41a**	Abortions. PMS. PTSD. pelvic infections
Infertility	85b	Erectile Disfunction (ED)
Infertility	120b	Miscarriages. Premature Births
Infertility	72a*	Low Sperm.
Infertility	64a	Low Sperm. Dry Cough
Infertility	173a	Vaginal Bleeding.
Infertility	136a	Genital Infection
Infertility	139b	Renal and Urinary Disfunction
Infertility	171b	False Pregnancy. Vomitting. Digestion.
Infertility	173a	Uterus.
Infertility	183b	Chronic Cough. Insomnia
Infertility	156a	Low Back. Genital Inflammation. Sore Muscle
Sex	129a	Eyes. Vaginal Bleeding. Low Platelet Count.
Sex	33a**	Frigidity. Mood Swings.
Sex	72a	Sexual Disorders
Sex	85b	Erectile Disfunction (ED)
Sex	60a	Low Libido
Sex	40b	Sexual Disorders
Sex	117a**	Syphillis. Gonorrhea.
Sex	152b	Gonorrhea
Sex	136a	Vaginal Infection
Sex	136b	Vaginal Infection
Sex	135a**	Irritation on Sexual Organs
Pain.Stress	74a	Cervical Plexus 2X
Pain	61b**	Neck 2X
Pain.Abdomen	94a	Pleural - Liver
Pain	49a	Cheekbone - Opposite Kidney
Pain.Joint	94b**	Cardiac - Adrenals
Pain.Stress	135b	Descending Colon - Rectum
Pain.Sex Organs	139a	Annexed 2X
Pain	147a	Renal Capsule 2X
Pain.Athletes Foot	180a**	Vena Cava 2X
Pain.Back	148a	Kidney 2X
Pain.Leg	155b	Cauda Equina 2X

Pain.Back	186b	Greater Sciatica Notch 2X
Skin	52b	Commissure 2x
Skin	54b	Tongue 2X
Skin	63a	1st Rib 2X
Skin	86a	Atrio Ventricular Node - Kidney
Skin	134b	Omentum 2X
Skin	138b	Appendix - Femoral Vein
Skin	135a**	Annexed 2X
Skin	126b	Brachial 2X
Skin	158a	Rectum 2X
Skin	187a**	Anus 2X
Skin	189a**	Ischial Ramus 2X
Skin	195a	Greater Trochaner (L) - Tensor Fascia Lata
Skin	195b**	Tensor Fascia Lata 2X
Skin	194b	Adductor 2X
Skin.anal	189a**	Ischium 2X
Infections. Hospitals. MRSA	139a**	Humerus 2X
Immune System	34b	
Hyperthyroidism	40a	Pituitary 2x
Sinusitis	42a	Frontal Sinus
Sinusitis	51b	Maxillary Sinus 2x
Sinusitis	45a	Eyelid upper 2x
Sinusitis	47a	Canthus Lateral 2x
Sinusitis	52a	Maxilla 2x
Sinusitis	50b	Ethmoid 2x
Sinusitis	51A	Nose 2x
Covid Sars	198a	Pes Anserine 2x

Specific Physical Issues

Brain Fog	62a	Parietal 2X
Brain Fog	48b	Circle of Willis 2X
Brain Fog	59b	Corpus Callosum (center) - Border Corpus Callusum (L)
Brain Fog	47b	Temple 2x
Brain Fog	71b	Thyroid - Medulla
Brain Fog	216b	Temporo Occipatal 2X
Tennis Elbow	81a	7th Cervical - 1st Thoracic
Carpal Tunnel	163a	Deltoid Insertion 2X
Cold Sores	56a	Tonsil 2X
Headaches	41a	Posthole 2x
Headaches	44a	Cranial 2x
Headaches	45b	Eyebrow2x
Headaches	57a	Malar 2X
Headaches	49b	Temple 2x
Headaches	58b	Maxillary Sinus 2X
Tinitus	52a	Circle of Willis 2X
Tinitus	66b	Inner Ear 2X
Teflon Pans	88a	Posterior Liver Lobe -Kidney
Gluten Intolerance	105a	Pancreas Head - Adrenals
Obesity	108b	Pancreas Body - Pancreas Tail
Food Allergies	105b	Pancreas Body - Stomach
Food Allergies - Sushi	108b	Pancreas Tail - Duodenum
Hot Tub - Pools	149b	Urethra - Urethra
Airplanes.Hotels.A/C	144a	T2 Verterbra 2X
Shoulder	203**	Bursa 2X
DDT.polio	163a	Quad - Quad
Pain. Neck. Fever. Arthritis	122b	C1 Verterbra-Pylorus
Pain. Back	151a	Quadratus Lumborum 2X
Pain relief	31a	Pain - Kidney
Back Pain	188b	Greater Sciatica Notch 2X
Back Pain	149b	Paravertebral 2X
Back Pain	156a	Sacrum 2X
Back Pain	192b	Greater Trochanter 2X
Pain. Muscle	27b	Corpus Callosum (center) - Border Corpus Callusum (L)
Pain. Muscle	64a	Temporal Lobe 2X

Pain. Muscle	70b	Medulla - Bladder
Pain. Muscle	114a	Pylorus - Tongue
Pain. Muscle	134a	Descending Colon - Liver
Pain. Muscle	175**	Armpit 2X
Pain. Muscle	147a	Renal Capsule 2X
Pain. Muscle	148a	Kidney 2X
Bloating	85**	Upper Liver 2x
Bloating	123a	Gall Bladder Duct - Kidney (R of L)
Yeast Infection	187**	Anus - Pylorus
Restless Leg	194b	Abductor 2X
Prevent Abortions	205**	External Knee - Quadratus Lumborum
Arthritis	205**	Plyacrticular Rheumatoid Arthritis
Surgery Scars	52a	Maxilla 2x
Surgery Scars	89b	Thymus- Rectum
Scarring. Breast Surgery	52**	Salivary Gland 2X
Scarring. Tonsillectomy	56b	Tonsil 2X
Scarring. Surgery	112**	Hospital Infections.
Light Sensitive/ Photosynthesis	212b	Systemic Lupus Erythematosus
Alchohol Detox	148a	Buzz Kill. gout
Fever	192b	Greater Trochanter 2X
Fever.Headache	191b	Achilles 2x
Balance	64a	Temporal 2x
Balance	69a	Medulla - Cerebellum
Balance	39b	Pole 2x
Balance	39a	Postpole 2X
Addiction/Detox	87b	Smokers. Shortness of Breath
Asthma	110**	Allergy.
PTSD.PMS	41a	Malnutrition. Abortions. Postpartum
Hospitals.	144a	T2 Vertebrae 2X
MRSA. Hospitals	164b	Hospital Infections.
Scarring. Surgery	131b	Hospital Infections.
Sleep	45b	Eye 2X
Sleep	44b	Eyebrow 2x
Sleep	/26**	Emotional Issues. Calcified Pineal Gland. Libido.
Sleep	28a	Brain Fog/Inflammation.Light.Irrationality

Sleep	65a	Eyes. Balance. Eating Disorder.
Sleep	64a	Headaches. Fever. Pyschosis. Muscle Ache. Skin
Sleep	48b	Eye. Optic Nerve. Dementia.
Sleep	69a	Balance. Dizziness.Depression. Headaches
Sleep	154a	Lower Limbs Paralysis. Digestine.Intolerance
Sleep	39a	Postpole 2X
Sleep	212a	Shallow Breathing.
Diet	58a	Weight Loss. Digestive Disorder.Thyroid
Fever	192b	Greater Trochanter 2X
Fever	191b	Achilles 2x
Coughing. Fever	180b	Vas Deferens - Larynx
Coughing	180a	Spermatic Cord 2 X
Coughing	144a	T2 Vertebra 2X
Coughing	190b	Popliteal 2X
Vomitting	70b	Medulla - Bladder
Vomitting	41b	Pituitary - Bladder
Vomitting	50a	Malar 2X
Vomitting	71**	Diaphragmatic Hiatus 2X
Vomitting	114b	Pylorus - Liver
Vomitting	113b	Pylorus 2X
Vomitting	114a	Pylorus - Tongue
Vomitting	108a	Pancreas - Liver
Vomitting	171b	Uterus 2X
Vomitting	155a	Douglas Sack (R,L) - Anterior Femoral Vein
Urinary Tract Infection	52a	Maxilla 2x
Urinary Tract Infection	172b	Uterus -Sacrum
Fever	192b	Greater Trochanter 2X
Fever	191b	Achilles 2X
Tinitus	66b	Inner Ear 2X
Gluten Intolerance	105a	Pancreas Head - Adrenals
Swimming	143b	Latissimus 2X
Athletes Foot	150b	Perirenal 2X
Athletes Foot	187**	Anus - Pylorus
Shingles	191b	Achilles 2x
Immune System	54a	Prearticular 2X
Immune System	160**	Appendix - Thymus

Rabies.Scar	219a	Scar - Armpit
Amputation	31b	Stump - Vertical & Horizontal
Diarrhea	41b	Pituitary - Bladder
Diarrhea	114b	Pylorus - Liver
Diarrhea	113b	Pylorus - Pylorus
Diarrhea	114a	Pylorus - Tongue
Diarrhea	105b	Pancreas - Stomach
Diarrhea	115b	Pylorus - Uterus
Diarrhea	133a	Transverse Colon - Bladder
Diarrhea	104b	Pancreas Head - Pylorus
Diarrhea	176b	Bladder - Anus
Menopause/Menstrual	89a	Thymus - Adrenals
Menopause	182a	Clitoris 2X
Menopause	181b	Ovary 2X
Menopause/Menstrual	189a	Ischium 2X
Menopause/Menstrual	161**	Kidney - Ureter
Menopause/Menstrual	33b	Pelvic Floor 2x
PTSD.PMS	41a	Pituitary - Ovary
Hernia	72**	Hiatus -Testicle or Vagina ®
Mold	47a	Canthus Lateral 2x
Mold	76**	Spleen 2X
Mold	185a	Upper Buttocks 2X
Mold	34b	Gallbladder 2x
Seizures.respiration.edemas	76b	3rd Cervical-Supraspinatus
Circulation. Blood Pressure. Digestion	73a	SCM 2X
Pain Neck. Elbow. Tennis elbow	77b	7th Cervical - 1st Thoracic
Nervous System. Seizure. paralysis	71a	Neck 2X
sore throat. Fever. headaches.nausea	82b	Manubrium 2X
Respiratory. Down pillows	83b	Pectoralis Major 2x
Nasal nose Sinusitis, ears, smell, detox	217 a	Bladder -Trauma
Breathing. SOB.	177b	Bacterial Reservoir

Prion Reservoir	36a	muscle control vaccines dementia	
Osteoporisis Bone	37b	hip joint inflammation	
Healthy Pregnancy	33b	Pelvic Floor 2x	
Kidney and Gall stones	34a	Scapula 2x	
Cosmetics. food	196a	Quad - Quad	
Sedentary. Inactive	126b	Belly Button 2x	

CHILDREN/ELDERLY

Learning	C	Pole 2x	39b
Self-Esteem. Negativity.	C	Glabella- medulla	42b
Shyness. Fear. Insecurity	C	Intercillary - Medulla	43a
ADHD Attention Deficit	C	Larynx 2X	71a
Tired. Haggard	C	Sigmoid - Rectum	140a
Childhood Cancer	C	Pleural 2X	93a
Learning Inability.Dyslexia	C	Pole 2x	39b
Stuttering. Speech	C	" "	39b
Lower Respiratory	C	Lacrimal 2X	44a
Bedwetting	C		
Hoof and Mouth Disease	C	Manubrium 2X	82b
Asphyxia. Respiratory	C	Aortic Knob - Th7	84b
Ear. Asthma. Digestive	C	Axilla - Axilla	161a
Cough. Phlem. Asphyxia	C	Pleural 2X	93b
Abdominal. Roseola	C	Hepatic Ligament - rt. Kidney	118b
Respiratory. Pneumonia	C	Pectoralis Major 2X	83b
Parkinson's Disease. False	E	Post Pineal - Medulla/Bladder	62a
Parkinson's Disease.	E	Kidney - Kidney	148a
Alzheimeir's	E	Femoral Fossa 2X	190a
Alzheimeir's	E	Temporal Lobe 2x	64a
Alzheimeir's	E	Wrist 2x	167a
Alzheimeir's	E	Calcaneus 2x	192a
Dementia	E	Prion Reservoir	36a
Dementia		Circle of Willis 2X	48b
Cold Feeling	E	Temporal Lobe 2x	64a
Balance	E	Pole 2x	39b
Eye Glaucoma	E	Canthus Lateral 2X	97a
Newborn Disease	E	Polyarticular Theumatoid Arthritis	210b

Low Energy. Back Pain	E	Cervical Plexus 2X	74a
Spleen Malfunction	E	Thymus - Rectum	89b
Respiratory. Renal bleeding	E	Urethra - Urethra	179b
Menopause	C/E	Menstrual Colic	89a
Menopause	E	Early Menopause. Excess hair.	133a
Menopause	E	Rectal Bleeding	181a
Menopause	E	Oral Ulcers. General	89a

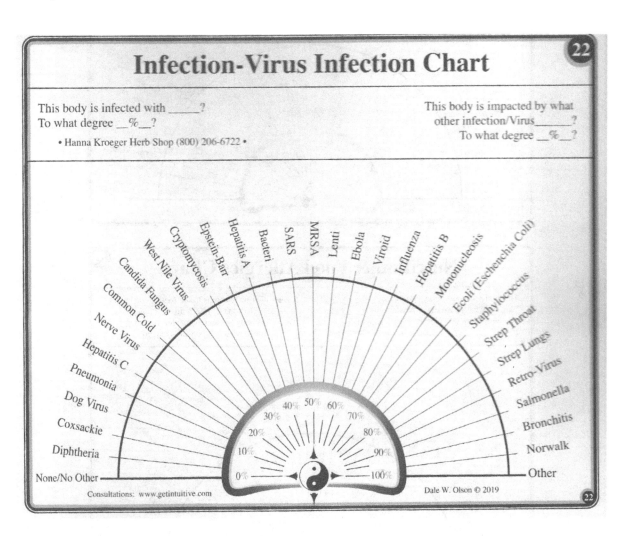

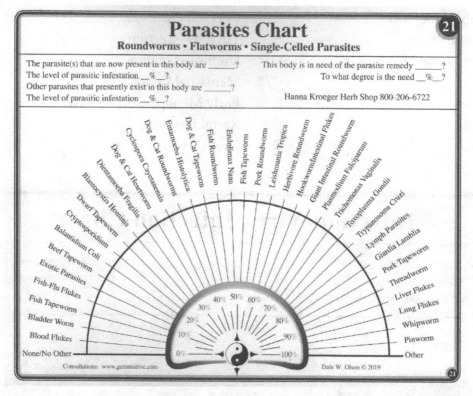

Parasites Chart
Roundworms • Flatworms • Single-Celled Parasites

The parasite(s) that are now present in this body are _____?
The level of parasitic infestation __%__?
Other parasites that presently exist in this body are _____?
The level of parasitic infestation __%__?

This body is in need of the parasite remedy _____?
To what degree is the need __%__?

Hanna Kroeger Herb Shop 800-206-6722

Consultations: www.getintuitive.com   Dale W. Olson © 2019

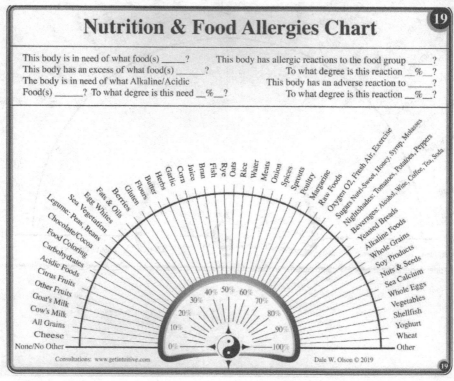

Nutrition & Food Allergies Chart

This body is in need of what food(s) _____?
This body has an excess of what food(s) _____?
The body is in need of what Alkaline/Acidic
Food(s) _____? To what degree is this need __%__?

This body has allergic reactions to the food group _____?
To what degree is this reaction __%__?
This body has an adverse reaction to _____?
To what degree is this reaction __%__?

Consultations: www.getintuitive.com   Dale W. Olson © 2019

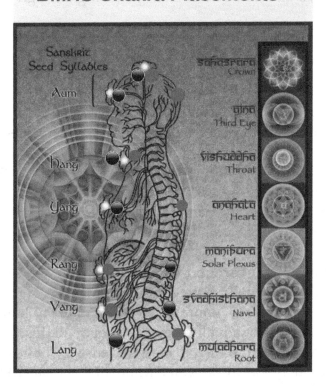

I use this Chakra clearing regularly at the start or end of a session as well as activating it for regular tune ups for myself and for loved ones. Try it during meditation and you'll feel the energy pulsing through you.

Dorothy Rowe:

"Chakras are energy organs or energy centers located in the body where very subtle and dense energies swirl together. There also exist sub chakras which reside between the seven main body chakras. Some energy healers identify hundreds of chakras, but for my work, I identify 6 earth chakras, 7 body chakras and 5 heaven chakras. The seven body chakras are most important for energy healing work."

Healing

Looking carefully at the crown chakra/root chakra axis. There is an energy form, like a vortex, circling above the head as well as below the pelvis. This swirling energy is a gentle massage which is both recognizing and enhancing the balance in these locations.

The crown and root chakras are coordinating with each other. The relationship between them is key to clearly appreciating the full evolutionary value of each stroke of human experience. Furthermore, Divine Dialogue is the mechanic from where this reality emerges. It is represented by two distinct flows of energy moving through the body, up and down.

Kundalini and Grace

Kundalini goes up (root to crown) and Grace flows down (crown to root).

Grace is present at every point of the creative process, and in every particle of creation. It brings the infinite potential of the subtle mechanics of manifestation to the body/mind system to the relative field of expression.

Kundalini moves earthy/earthly energy toward heaven. So it represents the refinement and deconstruction of the relative as it moves toward the qualitiless field of non manifest Source.

At the crown and root chakras, these two energies are balanced. This is because they are points of transition. One turns to become the other -hence, the swirling. This whirlpool energy also naturally maintains an openness where they are located. It also helps maintain suppleness, flexibility and connection to the whole range of life – from the unmanifest to the manifest.

Energetically, there is a point around the body where individuality ends and universality begins. To clarify, it is a point of reference where one is in transition between being isolated in space-time and being omnipresent. We could say that there is a gap at this precise spot. However, it is not a really a gap or spot at all. Instead, it is a feature of the field. It is actually a region within the range from dense to subtle of the field. This region is experiencing being energetically activated (more like massaged) by Being. There is also a gentle rocking motion as the whirlpool energy swirls around each node in the web of life. This is a very, very gentle process and it is carefully, lovingly exercised.

Increasing discernment

The light of pure perception is emerging from the gap. It is radiating into the area of self which we deem personal – your personal space. With the light comes improved personal perception. At the same time, there is clear intention behind this radiance. It is aimed at providing the resources for intelligently affecting healthy growth, increased energy, discernment. And as the light continues to penetrate the manifest levels of self, it brings silence. The silence in its full value seems to be preceding something.

Waiting… (rocking feeling still present)… Devic intelligence are receiving what looks like a boon of some sort. Going in for a finer look. They are receiving countless blessings from the region of the causal body responsible for wisdom archives. An ongoing relationship is establishing between the body's devic intelligence and the source of all body wisdom. Now, something very interesting is happening. The devic intelligence is receiving a formula for improved functioning. Furthermore, there is a family healing taking place in the field of devic intelligence. It turns out that the wisdom archives are actually the origin of the body's devic intelligence. There was, for a long time, some separation between individual body wisdom and cosmic body wisdom. However, the body wisdom is now clearly understanding the precise mode of functioning required to maintain ideal relations with its origin.

*In this healing, I am referring to very, very small packages of intelligence in the body. Ones that are responsible for maintenance and support of the physical.

Higher state of functioning

It feels like a holy family reunion. To clarify, it starts of course with reverence, but becoming much more than just recognition and acceptance. Something that looks like an initiation is taking place. And the acceptance is more of an inculcation into an order of greatness. This order of greatness (Eternal Order of Wisdom) has always existed. It has always been the origins of body wisdom. However, this degree of recognition has not been previously recognized. I honestly feel that it's the increased intelligence and discernment which made the body wisdom worthy of this higher state of functioning. From a practical level, this includes healing rites. The body intelligence will purify the body according to cosmic cycles of daily, (approximately) bi-monthly, annually and larger cycles. Furthermore, there will be times of deep silence where the light of pure perception will continue to expand its presence. It will promote targeted upgrades in the areas of the body most in need. The relationship between body wisdom and cosmic wisdom will reveal itself through synchronicities. This will lead to greater success in action, faster fulfillment of intentions, and improvement in relationship with oneself".

Heavy Metal Toxin and Mold Placements

In 2005 the Chief Scientist of NASA presented a slide show about Future of Warfare where nanoparticulate bio sensors would be released through aerosol spraying. Geoengineering is the aerosol spraying of chemicals and toxins in micro nano particulate matter that enters the body and goes through the blood brain barrier. Among the many toxins sprayed on us all like bugs are aluminum, strontium and barium. The Heavy Metal clearing protocols listed below will help mitigate and lift the heavy metals. This scan should be done regularly on all since everyone around the world is regularly being bombarded with aerosol sprays as well as being uptaken in our food and water supplies.

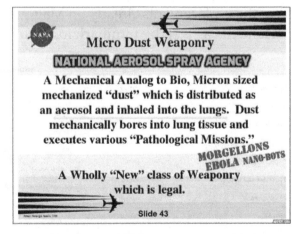

Geoengineering is the aerosol spraying of our skies on a regular basis now. Please refer to my book, *"Geoengineering aka Chemtrails"* where I list hundreds and hundreds of

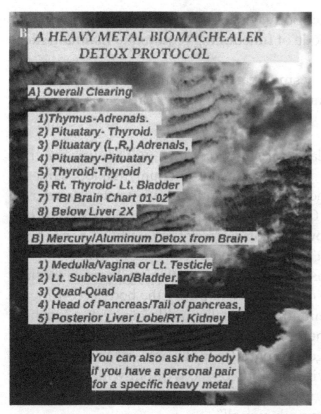

A HEAVY METAL BIOMAGHEALER DETOX PROTOCOL

A) Overall Clearing

1) Thymus-Adrenals.
2) Pituatary- Thyroid.
3) Pituatary (L,R,) Adrenals,
4) Pituatary-Pituatary
5) Thyroid-Thyroid
6) Rt. Thyroid- Lt. Bladder
7) TBI Brain Chart 01-02
8) Below Liver 2X

B) Mercury/Aluminum Detox from Brain -

1) Medulla/Vagina or Lt. Testicle
2) Lt. Subclavian/Bladder.
3) Quad-Quad
4) Head of Pancreas/Tail of pancreas,
5) Posterior Liver Lobe/RT. Kidney

You can also ask the body if you have a personal pair for a specific heavy metal

patents for weather modification since 1920!. Micro-sized nanobots that get past the blood brain barrier are now regularly sprayed across the world where a disease from this spraying, called "Moregellons Disease" has been discovered. Issues related to heavy metal toxic spraying include fatigue, respiratory and many Covid, Flu like symptoms. Regular scanning and clearing should be done as a standard protocol.

Coding

Coding is an exciting new protocol with full credit to Mr. Daniel Blair for the inspiration and work up to possibly use codes to implement specific issue healing. The idea is that the code encompasses several BiomagHealing placements with a code. One then can set the intention of the placements that have been set on the Mannequin by activating the Code Number only and the needed placements will be set. Again, it is our INTENTION that activates, so coding is still in its trial phases, but is promising. Codes were determined by muscle testing. I have these placements already on Maggy the Mannequin. You may possibly activate these placements as well by familiarizing yourself with the placements of the group and then

MOST COMMON PATHOGENS CODING	
YERSINIA PESTIS	98N98
RABIES	6768P
TUBERCULOSIS	LD558
IMMUNE SYSTEM/GUT	586J5
PSUEDO AUREGONOSA	589H
EPSTEIN BARR VIRUS	98676
LYME DISEASE	6858H
MALARIA	56506
PATHOGEN VIRUS	DG68
PATHOGEN BACTERIA	E668
PATHOGEN FUNGUS	858R
PATHOGEN PARASITE	8F68

ISSUES AND SYMPTOMS CODING 2	
PAIN	2D2B2
BACK PAIN	B44B4
INFLAMATION	B115B
CANCER	CC231
HOSPITAL SCAR/MRSA	444B4
BREAST SURGERY/SCARRING	2P641
OBESITY	D2432
TOOTH ACHE	FGE4
ADDICTION/DETOX	AAB24
DIABETES	2B132A4

ISSUES AND SYMPTOMS CODING	
TERRAIN TOXIC CLEARING (heavy metal, mold, Covid Virus)	A13369
HEAVY METAL	54
MOLD	LRS3
INSOMNIA	2B463B
FATIGUE	4L54
BRAIN FOG	H44RS
HEADACHES/BALANCE	1A2A2
Emotions	R688
ROCKACHAKRA	84PG
CHAKRA CLEARING/ACTIVATING	6R38T
ELDERLY	G65G
CHILDREN	BB11
RESERVOIR CLEARING	EEJ36
FLU/COMMON COLD	TLD668
VACCINE INJURIES	CCC44

set you activation with intention. Muscle test to see if you have been effective. If we are successful with this coding technique we may be able to effectively activate placements of groups of people at a distance. What a world THAT would be!

1) Muscle test to find what Code and/or group of symptoms you wish to address. 2) Ask if this code can help the soul you are wishing to activate placements? (You may also ask if this code can be applied to a group of individuals as well). 3) Visually, if possible, look at the individual placements in the code, if not ask if you can activate the needed placements in that code? 4) If yes, activate the code number with your intention to activate the appropriate and corresponding placements in that code. 5) Ask is follow up is needed?

I have found that I can prove that the coding is successful with "provable" results like better night sleeps if I activated the Insomnia code # 28463B or for a toothache # FGE4 or ???. Also, reservoir clearing is also handy for beginning and ending session work.

"You Don't Get Old You Get Mold" ~ Dr. Robert Young

Mold is one of the most prolific of issues and ailments we have today. Mold is found in homes, in our foods and in the air. Exposure to mold can cause several health issues such as; throat irritation, nasal stuffiness, eye irritation, cough, and wheezing, as well as skin irritation in some cases. Exposure to mold may also cause heightened sensitivity depending on the time and nature of exposure. Exposure to mold can cause several health issues such as; throat irritation, nasal stuffiness, eye irritation, cough, and wheezing, as well as skin irritation in some cases. Exposure to mold may also cause heightened sensitivity depending on the time and nature of exposure. Mold is also known to cause asthma and life-threatening primary and secondary infections in immune-compromised patients that have been exposed. Toxic mold exposure has also been linked to more serious, long-term effects like memory loss, insomnia, anxiety, depression, trouble concentrating, and confusion.

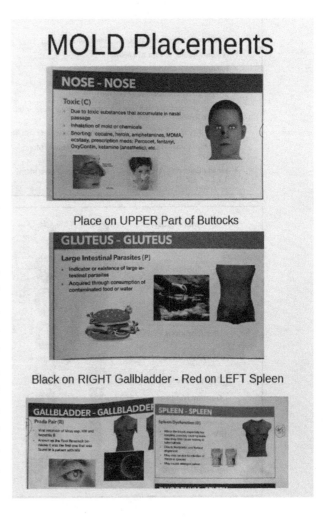

If you find someone who has mold, ask is it airborne or food borne? Then, ask if mold is present in their home? And if that is the cause of their mold issues? Then, find where the mold in the house may be located by scanning. Is it in their kitchen? Bedroom, bath? Etc. Then ask, Is is on the right side or left? High or low? And find the effecting mold for them to discover and replace.

Lyme Disease is caused by only .5% due to tick bites. Full scanning to find the causal effects of so-called Lyme Disease is essential. Like Fibromyalgia and many other misdiagnosed diseases, Lyme's has many issues caused by several different issues including Tuberculosis.

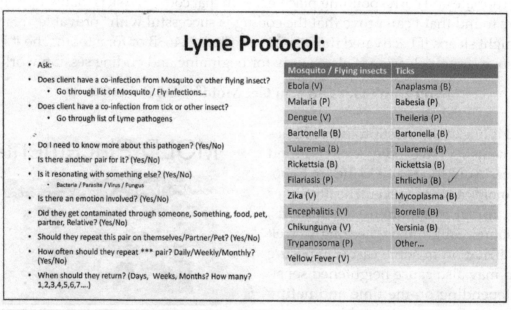

Lyme Protocol:

- Ask:
- Does client have a co-infection from Mosquito or other flying insect?
  - Go through list of Mosquito / Fly infections...
- Does client have a co-infection from tick or other insect?
  - Go through list of Lyme pathogens

- Do I need to know more about this pathogen? (Yes/No)
- Is there another pair for it? (Yes/No)
- Is it resonating with something else? (Yes/No)
  - Bacteria / Parasite / Virus / Fungus
- Is there an emotion involved? (Yes/No)
- Did they get contaminated through someone, Something, food, pet, partner, Relative? (Yes/No)
- Should they repeat this pair on themselves/Partner/Pet? (Yes/No)
- How often should they repeat *** pair? Daily/Weekly/Monthly? (Yes/No)
- When should they return? (Days, Weeks, Months? How many? 1,2,3,4,5,6,7....)

Mosquito / Flying insects	Ticks
Ebola (V)	Anaplasma (B)
Malaria (P)	Babesia (P)
Dengue (V)	Theileria (P)
Bartonella (B)	Bartonella (B)
Tularemia (B)	Tularemia (B)
Rickettsia (B)	Rickettsia (B)
Filariasis (P)	Ehrlichia (B) ✓
Zika (V)	Mycoplasma (B)
Encephalitis (V)	Borrelia (B)
Chikungunya (V)	Yersinia (B)
Trypanosoma (P)	Other...
Yellow Fever (V)	

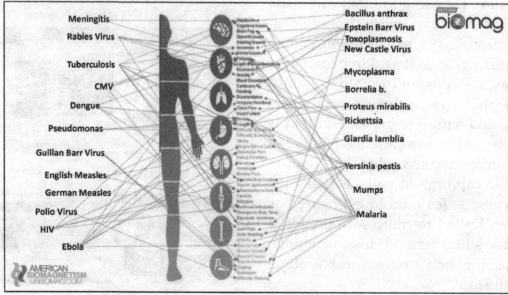

New Frontiers of Biomagnetism

Animal magnetism refers to how they orient themselves using Earth's magnetic field. It would make sense that to counter an insect's magnetic biology, opposing magnets may disrupt their fields and keep them from attacking. Dr. Garcia has found many, many issues and symptoms to common illness' related to the mosquito as seen in this chart he designed for placements for mosquito bites and infections.

Mosquitos carry many, many diseases and are a cause of many symptoms diagnosed incorrectly. The mosquito infection scan protocol should be of standard protocol for regular session work. Also, mosquito season is also extending so regular scanning should be done.

MOSQUITO ACQUIRED INFECTIONS:

- Ebola
  - (Arch of foot / Arch of foot) &
  - (Anterior costal Right / Anterior costal left)
- Bartonella
  - Cardiac sphincter / Appendix
  - Vagina / Descending Colon (Dr. G)
  - Cervical Vertebrae 3 / Vagina (Dr. G)
- Malaria (Most Common Pathogens sheet)
- PseudoMalaria = Haemoproteus (Dr. G)
  - Bladder/ Scapula Left, LADCA/Vagina,
  - Bladder / Lumbar 4, Bladder/Vagina
- Dengue Virus (Pituitary / Bladder)
- Dengue "Hemorrhagic" (Medulla / Bladder)
- Zika Virus (Anterior Left Costal / Left Kidney)
- Yellow Fever Virus (Pancreatic Ligament / Descending Colon)

- Chikungunya Virus (Descending Colon / Anus)
- Eastern Equine Encephalitis (Cerebellum / SCM Left)
- Tularemia (Francisella tularensis) (Thymus / Pineal)
- Rickettsia (Wrists, Calcaneous, Temporal Lobes)
- Lymphatic Filariasis (Mastoide / Mastoides
- Western Equine Encephalitis (Bladder / Adrenal) (Dr. G)
- Heart worm ?
- *Dirofilaria (Dog heartworm)?*
- French heartworm?
- West Nile Virus ???
- Q Fever *Coxiella burnetii ?*

Putting magnets around your one wrist and your neck prevents mosquito bites according to this article!

"Why Magnets may Repel Mosquitoes and other Predatory Insects
Thesis'Theory in Practice" ~ Stephen Verdon, Ph.D

"The presence of the magnet elicited a distinct reaction from Mosquitoes –they dart away from it. To determine the strength of this repugnant force, we examined the results with several other people who were 'covered' with Mosquitoes from Head to Toe. It appears that the only person in our experimental group that was not being 'Eaten Alive' was Michael Saxon (Field Researcher) who was the only person wearing magnets around his neck and wrist.

This is a condition commonly known as 'Tonic Immobility' or a Temporary Paralysis that naturally occurs when Mosquitoes are disrupted before they bite. Sure enough, the magnets repelled the Mosquitoes with surprising results. Why the intense reaction? The apparent interaction between Atmospheric Static Electricity and Magnetically Charged Magnemax 'Earths-Core' Magnets produces a weak but notable electromagnetic field. When a Mosquito comes close to that field, it seems to disrupt the Mosquitoes Sixth-Sense aka Electroreception. Many species of Mosquitoes have sensory receptors that detect minute changes of electricity in the air. These electrical impulses originate and are carried through Atmospheric Ions.

Mosquitoes are literally wired for hunting. These predators are equipped with a special sense known as Electroreception which allows them to home in on their prey with precise accuracy. Other members of the Mosquito family also share this trait but the Common Mosquitoes Electroreception (Electroreceptive animals use this sense to locate objects around them) are the extremely finely tuned. Electroreception is used in electrolocation (detecting objects) and for electrocommunication. Electroreception simply means the ability to detect Electrical or Magnetic currents.

What does electricity have to do with Mosquitoes? Any muscular movement or twitches in living animals create a small electrical current. At hospitals, electrocardiogram machines track the electricity resulting from our heartbeat. Bees for example, collect a positive static charge while flying through the air (see Atmospheric electricity). When a bee visits a flower, the charge deposited on the flower takes a while to leak away into the ground. Bees can detect both the presence and the pattern of electric fields on flowers and use this information to know if a flower has been recently visited by another bee and is therefore likely to have a reduced concentration of pollen.

The mechanism of electric field reception in animals living in the air like bees is based on mechano-reception, not electroreception. Bees receive the electric field changes via the Johnston's organs in their antennae and possibly other mechano-receptors. They distinguish different temporal patterns and learn them. During the waggle dance, Honeybees appear to use the electric field emanating from the dancing bee for distance communication.

These electrical impulses originate and are carried through Atmospheric Ions. Open air does not conduct this electricity away from our bodies, but for Mosquitoes it does. Ions are particles that have an electrical charge because they have lost or gained an electron. Static Electricity is easily transported by Humidity. You can compare this to how batteries work. It's set up like an electro chemical cell that separates negative from positively charged ions".

BiomagHealing Head Placements

The medical community has known for years that biomagnetic protocols promote the healing process, particularly of bone fractures. For over 40 years many doctors have used pulsed biomagnetic therapy to support healing of fractures and have had a high rate of success. Several magnetic instruments have already been FDA-approved and sanctioned for both safety and therapeutic implications. The success of this therapy is attributed, in part, to its facilitating the migration of calcium ions and osteoblasts to heal broken bones in less than the usual time. In addition, the migration of calcium occurs away from joints to reduce painful arthritic joint inflammation. The result is the noninvasive promotion of natural healing, without the use of unnatural chemicals and drugs. Adequate magnetic energy also softens or eliminates scar tissue formed during the healing process. Pulsed biomagnetism does not deal with polarity magnetic healing but attempts to return the 'injured' cells back to health with pulsing.

Just these head placements alone can help alleviate and heal the many of the issues listed. Just learning these head placements by memory will help many (as long as you have magnets with you).

Head Magnet Placements Issues and Symptoms

Common cold * Fevers * Flu Symtpoms * Runny Nose * TMJ/ Lock Jaw, Insomnia, Fatigue * Respiratory * Shortness of Breath * MS * Rashes * Diarrhea * Mold * Tooth Pain * Bleeding Gums * Shortness of Breath *Headaches *Tinitus *Sleep/Insomnia *Brain Fog * Nose Bleeds * Halitosis * Facial Paralysis * Eye Strain/Vision *Gluacoma * Cataracts *Balance *Childhood Learning Slowness * Dyslexia * ADHD * Dementia * Vomitting * Anorexia * Sex Appetite * Inflammation * Muscle Pain * Bronchitis * Laryngitis * Breast Lymphatic Issues * Trauma * Mononucleoisis * Self-Esteem * Drug Addiction * Excess Emotions * Insecurity *Digestion *Nerves *Numbness * Anger * Loss of Humor * Brain Fog * Anxiety * Depression * Panic Attacks * Aggression * Fear * Irritability * Lonliness * Moody * Suicidal * Inspiration * Intuition * Pineal Gland Cleansing * Elderly Temperature Control *

Brain Scan Charts

This is Dr. Garcia's proprietary brain scan chart he developed. He is able to greatly reduce injuries from concussions, brain inflammation as well as physical issues associated and located in the brain using this chart.

I start by scanning the middle numbers nose to back (Nz-Iz) and then ask if there is a pair or and individual placement? Red and/or black? Once you locate a placement(s) scan and drill down to find what part of the body is associated and whether red or black placement is needed. Dr. Garcia developed this chart and protocol to assist in relieving Traumatic Brain Injuries or TBI. Go to the Biomag Bible after you have looked up issues and ailments in Appendix II. The page number is listed for the placement for each issue around the head listed here. Make sure to muscle test for correctness of placements and if further placements are needed for this specific issue.

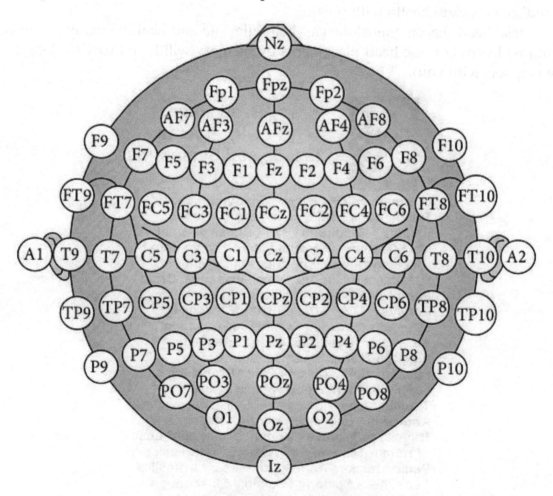

You can further drill down to where in the brain issues need placements for. Remember the more focused and the more you drill down to the exact causal factors (by muscle testing), the better your results will be. So I just ask of the 12 cranial nerves.."are their any here that will help the soul I'm working with now..?" If yes, I scan and place. Then scan again and again until I get an all done or clear.

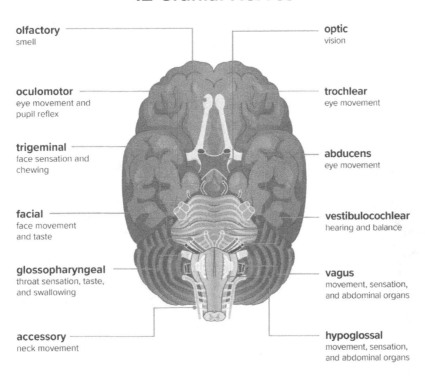

MEDICAL**NEWS**TODAY

12 Cranial Nerves

olfactory
smell

oculomotor
eye movement and
pupil reflex

trigeminal
face sensation and
chewing

facial
face movement
and taste

glossopharyngeal
throat sensation, taste,
and swallowing

accessory
neck movement

optic
vision

trochlear
eye movement

abducens
eye movement

vestibulocochlear
hearing and balance

vagus
movement, sensation,
and abdominal organs

hypoglossal
movement, sensation,
and abdominal organs

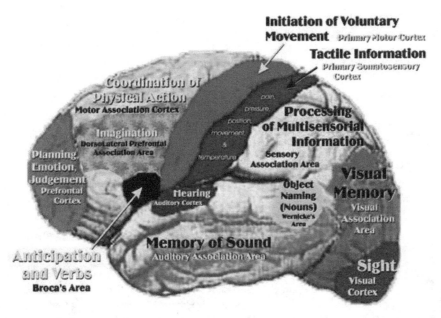

Initiation of Voluntary Movement Primary Motor Cortex

Tactile Information Primary Somatosensory Cortex

Coordination of Physical Action Motor Association Cortex

pain, pressure, position, movement & temperature

Processing of Multisensorial Information

Imagination DorsoLateral Prefrontal Association Area

Sensory Association Area

Planning, Emotion, Judgement Prefrontal Cortex

Hearing Auditory Cortex

Object Naming (Nouns) Wernicke's Area

Visual Memory Visual Association Area

Anticipation and Verbs Broca's Area

Memory of Sound Auditory Association Area

Sight Visual Cortex

Concept by: Silvia Helena Cardoso, PhD
Center for Biomedical Information, University of Campinas, Brazil

Brain Map Review — Wizard of Ads Academy

Spinal Column Nerve Root Issues

Another effective scanning technique is to drill down to find what nerves and associated symptoms are being impacted. Start with the Verterbrae and go right to left until you find the symptoms associated with the specific vertebrae and nerve. Once you find the nerve root keep drilling down to the right through muscle testing to find the symptoms and set your intention on the vertebrae placements. Ask if the corresponding placements are vertical or horizontal.

You can bring up very specific anatomy charts of ligaments, nerves, veins, bones, muscles, etc. to find where the exact placement(s) are needed.

VERTEBRAL LEVEL	NERVE ROOT*	INNERVATION	POSSIBLE SYMPTOMS
C1	C1	Intracranial Blood Vessels	Headaches • Migraine Headaches
	C2	• Eyes • Lacrimal Gland	• Dizziness • Sinus Problems
C2		• Parotid Gland • Scalp	• Allergies • Head Colds • Fatigue
	C3	• Base of Skull • Neck	• Vision Problems • Runny Nose
C3	C4	Muscles • Diaphragm	• Sore Throat • Stiff Neck
C4	C5	• Neck Muscles • Shoulders	• Cough • Croup • Arm Pain
C5	C6	• Elbows • Arms • Wrists	• Hand and Finger Numbness
C6	C7	• Hands • Fingers • Esopha-	or Tingling • Asthma • Heart
	C8	gus • Heart • Lungs • Chest	Conditions • High Blood Pressure
C7	T1		
T1	T2	Arms • Esophagus	Wrist, Hand and Finger
	T3	• Heart • Lungs • Chest	Numbness or Pain • Middle Back
T2		• Larynx • Trachea	Pain • Congestion • Difficulty
T3	T4		Breathing • Asthma • High Blood
T4	T5	Gallbladder • Liver	Pressure • Heart Conditions
T5	T6	• Diaphragm • Stomach	• Bronchitis • Pneumonia
T6	T7	• Pancreas • Spleen	• Gallbladder Conditions
T7	T8	• Kidneys • Small Intestine	• Jaundice • Liver Conditions
T8	T9	• Appendix • Adrenals	• Stomach Problems • Ulcers
T9	T10		• Gastritis • Kidney Problems
T10	T11	Small Intestines • Colon • Uterus	
T11	T12	Uterus • Colon • Buttocks	
T12	L1		
L1	L2	Large Intestines	Constipation • Colitis • Diarrhea
L2		• Buttocks • Groin	• Gas Pain • Irritable Bowel
L3	L3	• Reproductive Organs	• Bladder Problems • Menstrual
	L4	• Colon • Thighs • Knees	Problems • Low Back Pain
L4	L5	• Legs • Feet	• Pain or Numbness in Legs
L5	SACRAL	Buttocks • Reproductive Organs • Bladder • Prostate Gland • Legs • Ankles • Feet • Toes	Constipation • Diarrhea • Bladder Problems • Menstrual Problems • Lower Back Pain • Pain or Numbness in Legs

Emotional Placements

Emotional issues are the causal root of 80-90% of all our physical issues and ailments. So finding the emotional causes and then drill down to specific placement for those emotions are essential to overall health and well-being.

Also, when scanning for emotions, the issues brought up may be coming to them from another person, (i.e. boss who hates them, partner issues laid on them, etc.). You can also muscle scan to find when these issues began (previous life, youth, 20's, 30,'s etc.,) Drill down to find exact year to help them focus and recall.

This work is like peeling an onion. You drill down to peel layers and layers of issues, so you keep scanning and asking are there more placements needed today? Over and over and over again until you get a "no more" by muscle testing.

Way to Scan for Emotional Issues?

1. Dr. Garcia's Emotions List
2. Emotion Codes Scan Sheet
3. Souls related Emotions

Does this soul have emotional issues associated with this physical issue (be specific!)?

If Yes, then do Emotional Scan sheet

1. Is the emotional issue associated with any physical issues on this scan sheet?
2. If in column or number "___", is it an odd number? Even number? (remember, it can be several emotional issues and when brought up can trigger more emotional recalls!)
3. In What Page? Or Column "___"?, Number "____"?.

Emotional Placing

Once you've identified an emotion, then ask, is there emotional issues attached to this physical location?

a. When was this emotion attained?
b. Was it by them, or brought on to them?
c. Will a magnetic pair placement help them at this time?
d. Where does the placement go?
e. Will this person need to release this emotion to heal?
f. Do they need to meditate? To forgive? To let go? etc.
f. Will they need a follow up to this session? If so when?
g. Do they need to do follow up placements? If so, for how long?

This is another scan emotional chart you can locate emotional issues. Start at center to find specific emotions. Then go back to body scan to find where to do the correct placements.

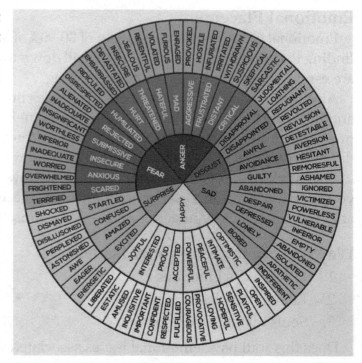

1. You may ask the soul if they can relate to the issues you found?

2. Are there more physical issues associated with this emotions?

3. Does this soul need to address these emotional issues?

4. Then ask if meditating, forgiveness, confronting, etc. is necessary to alleviate emotional issue affecting the body.

5. Command the body to release the negative emotions.

6. You may/can ask is these issues are something they brought on, or was brought onto them by outside souls and issues?

7. You may ask if there are more emotional issues that need to be addressed in this session today?

8. You may/can ask if this person has effectively dealt with/let go of this emotional baggage causing physical ailments? Then you may wish to ask them to meditate and reflect on the issues affecting them to get clear.

9. Then scan and ask, are there any friends or family members who may have contracted similar issues? Or can any other family members benefit from these placements today? If yes, set your intention to place magnets on that named person(s)

IF these are deep and highly sensitive issues, be sensitive to this. Some become highly embarrassed and protective when their innermost thoughts and feelings are brought out loud. Yet, many times I have experienced a deep sense of relief to be able to verbalize the emotions trapped inside the soul's body.

Once emotional scan I did for a soul came back "rape, torment, trauma, etc." When I told her what I found she became very distraught and upset that a stranger was able to bring up her childhood rape and torture that she had not told anyone else before. I asked to do a follow up session and she declined. Weeks later she lost her job and got in a car accident on the same day. Related? We don't know, but be respectful, always!

I scan this sheet for 1) basic emotions or 2) For specific emotion(s) for a specific ailment or issue. To find the emotion I ask first "is it in column A-E? Then, when I find the column I ask which number box on the left hand column 1-9? Let's say I find column C-3 now of the 5 in the box which one is it 1-5? So if I got #4 in the box…

C-3.5..the emotion would be Insanity emotion. Then ask if it is current? Coming from them? Or at them? ect. There are over 440 emotions listed here to scan for. If emotions cause 80% + of our physical issues, then this scan sheet is a must for optimal healing.

EMOTIONS

	A	B	C	D	E
1	Abandonment	Deobligationi	Hyper sensibility	Non-Compliance	Sleeplessness
	Absence	Depression	Hysteria	Nostalgia	Sorrow
	Abuse	Derision	Impartiality	Nuisance	Spirituality/Religious
	Accusation	Despair	Impatience	Obsession	Stagnation
	Addiction	Desperation	Impotence	Overprotection	Stress
2	Affliction	Disappointment	Impression	Overwhelmed	Suffering
	Affliction	Discrimination	Incomprehension	Pain	Superstition
	Aggression	Disenchantment	Incongruity	Panic	Suspicion
	Agony	Disgust	Inconsideration	Paranoia	Tedium
	Agressiveness	Dishonesty	Inconsistency	Paranormal	Temper
3	Ambition	Disillusion	Indecision	Passion	Tenacity
	Anger	Dislike	Indifference	Perfectionism	Tension
	Anguish	Disorganization	Infatuation	Persecution	Terror
	Annoyance	Disown	Injustice	Pessimism	Threaten
	Anorexia	Distrust	Insanity	Physical Integrity	Tiredness
4	Anxiety	Dread	Integrity	Pressure	Torment
	Apathy	Economy	Intimacy	Pride	Torture
	Asphyxia	Enthusiasm	Intimidation	Pride	Transition
	Avarice	Envy	Intolerance	Procrastination	Trauma
	Bankruptcy	Erotism	Intuition	Punishment	uncertainty
5	Bashfulness	Exclusion	Irresponsibility	Rage	Unconsciousness
	Betrayal	Exhaustion	Irritability	Reconciliation	Undefensive
	Bias	Exile	Isolation	Reconsideration	Ungrateful
	Bitterness	Expectative	Jealousy	Regret	Unhappiness
	Blackmailing	Extravagance	Justification	Rejection	unproductive
6	Boredom	Failure	Lack of interest	Repression	Unprotection
	Censored	Fanaticism	Lack of love	Reprimand	Vanity
	Claustrophobia	Fantasy	Lack of reo	Repugnance	Vengeance
	Comparison	Fatigue	Laziness	Resentment	Violation
	Complex	Fear	Libido	Responsibility	Violence
7	Concerns	Fearfulness	Loneliness	Restlessness	Weariness
	Conflict	Finances	Longing	Ridiculous	Whim
	Confrontation	Fright	Loss	Rumor	Will
	Confusion	Frustration	Lying	Sadness	Xenophobia
	Contradiction	Gluttony	Maleficence	Self Punishment	
8	Cowardliness	Gossiping	Mediocrity	Self-esteem	
	Creativity	Grief	Melancholy	Selfishness	
	Crisis	Guilt	Misplacement	Senselessness	
	Criticism	Harassment	Morality	Sensuality	
	Cruelty	Harm	Mourning	Sexuality	
9	Crying	Harmony	Necessity	Shameless	
	Deceit	Hate	Negation	Shameless	
	Decrease	Horror	Negativity	Shock	
	Delirium	Humbleness	Negligence	Shyness	
	Demotivation	Hungry	Negotiation	Silence	

Ask for: kinesiology, first, second or third person.

If there is any doubt, ask if it is excess or lack of it.

The emotional stressors may be represented by an event, a no event, an emotion, a mood or a feeling or as a trigger or a result.

Emotional Placements.

	Pg. #	Pairs
Panic Attack. Nervous breakdown	68b	Cerebellum 2x
Moody		Atlas 2X
Bipolar.Depression.Fatigue	68a	Occipital 2X
Dependence on Mother	230b	Belly Button-Testicle
Dependence on Father	221b	Belly Button-Uterus
Moral Integrity. Lying.	223a	Post Pineal 2X
Superiority Complex	222a	Central Sulcus 2X
Inspiration	224a	Sylvian Fissure 2X
Arrogance. Pride.	224**	Adrenal - Liver
Lust	222a	Pineal - Prostrate/Uterus
Anger. Rights Violated	230a	Liver-Heart
Gluttony. Obesity	229a	Stomach-Heart
Jealousy	232**	Atlas - Uterus
Jealousy	226a	Heart - Pancreas
Laziness. Fatigue. fear	196b	Patella 2X
Laziness. Lack of Caring	228a	Spleen - Hypothalmus
Cruelty. Hate	225a	Medula - Heart
Impatience. Always Feel Rushed	227a	Thymus - Ovary/Testicle
Doubt. Uncertainty	232b	Back of Hand 2X
Guilt. Remorse	228a	Lung 2X
Intolerance. Attention Deficit	227b	Trachea - Heart
Depression	60a	Pineal 2X
Depression	68a	Occipital 2X
Depression	98a	Pancreatic Duct - Kidney (L)
Depression	138a	Appendix - Pleura
Depression. Sadness	68a	Occipital - Occipital
Depression. Sadness	228b	Lung - Medulla
Depression. Sadness. guilt.	223b	Post Pineal - Cerebral Amygdala
Depression. Suicide. Lupus	212b	Systemic Lupus Erythematosus
Materialism	230b	Transversal Colon-Ovary/Testicle
Anger	62a	Parietal 2X
Anger	64a	Temporal 2X
Anger	112b	Peri-Pancreatic 2X
Hate. Anger	221b	Cerebral Amygdala-Thymus
Evil. Hatred.	224b	Occipital -Testicle

Loneliness	221a	Hippocampus - Cerebral Amygdala
Stress	74a	Cervical Plexus 2X
Stress	40a	Pituitary 2x
Stress. Panic Attacks. Nervous	100b	Stomach 2X
Stress	135a	Descending Colon - Rectum
Stress	155b	Cauda Equina 2X
Stress. Fear of Flying	114a	Pylorus -Tongue
Anxiety. Fear	64a	Temporal Lobe 2X
Anxiety. Fear	44b	Eyebrow2x
Anxiety. Fear	161a	Axilla 2x
Anxiety. Fear	196b	Patella 2X
Fear. Insecurity. Shyness	43a	Interciliary - Medula
Trauma	219	Bladder - Trauma Zone
Trauma	219	Kidney (L) - Trauma Zone
Trauma	219	Kidney (R) - Trauma Zone
Trauma. tissue repair	217	Acute Trauma = Maria Pair
Trauma	217	Temporal - I or Salva Pair
		ct. Mandible. descending colon. Vena cava rt. scapula rt.
Loss	.	
Sex Disorder	40a	Pituitary 2x
Emotional Disorders	42b	Glabella-Medulla
Psychiatric Issues	59b	Corpus Callosum Center- CC L border
Delirium	112a	Pancreatic Ligament-Desc. Colon
Mental Shift	126b	Belly Button 2x
Unresolved Emotional issues	128a	Duodenum-Spleen

Teeth Issues Are Critical to Optimal Biomag Healing

Many issues can be traced and followed from the teeth. Below are nerves connected to body organs and nerves associated with different tooth/nerve ailments. Are you aware that studies show that over 80% of women who get breast cancer have had root canals.

Once you locate the tooth then drill down to the nerves associated with that tooth and find the corresponding organ or nerve placements down the body.

Then ask if the target cells are in the muscles, nerves, ligaments, artery, vein, bone or space between.

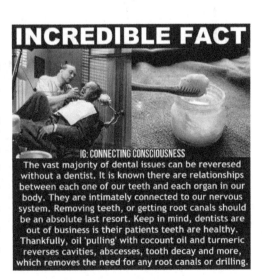

INCREDIBLE FACT

IG: CONNECTING CONSCIOUSNESS

The vast majority of dental issues can be reveresed without a dentist. It is known there are relationships between each one of our teeth and each organ in our body. They are intimately connected to our nervous system. Removing teeth, or getting root canals should be an absolute last resort. Keep in mind, dentists are out of business is their patients teeth are healthy. Thankfully, oil 'pulling' with cocount oil and turmeric reverses cavities, abscesses, tooth decay and more, which removes the need for any root canals or drilling.

It is also know now that over 80% of women who develop breast cancer also have had root canal surgery! Use the charts below to find the placements for tooth issues and associated organs or other body parts or systems.

To drill down to issues you can use this handy chart or the teeth chart with associated nerves and organs below.

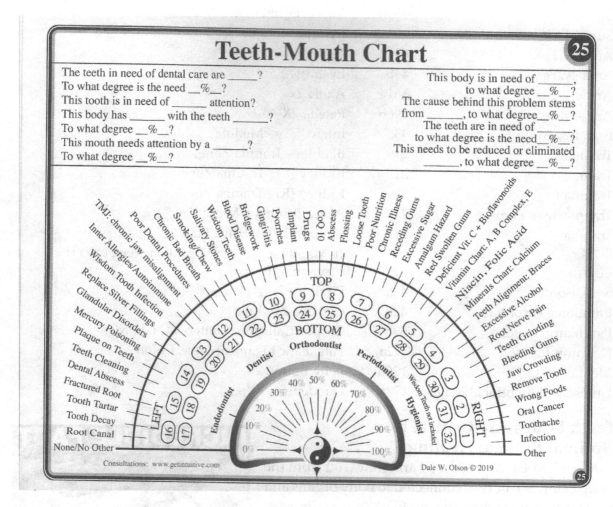

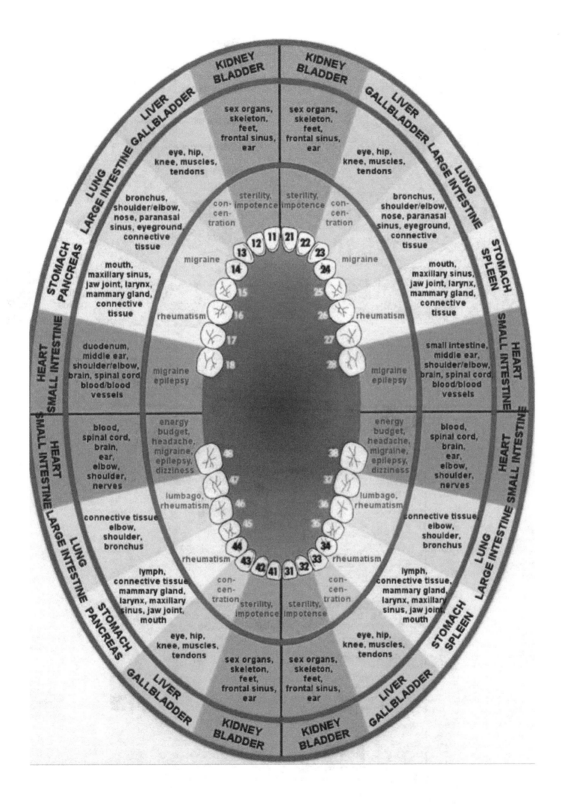

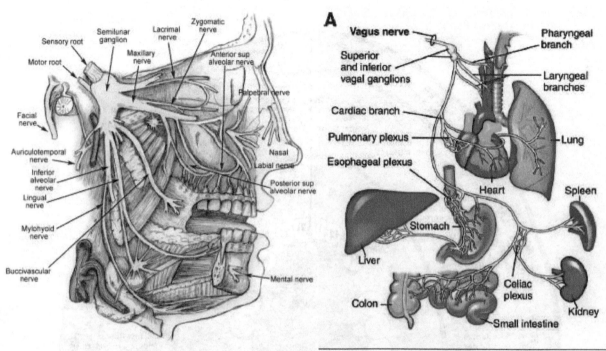

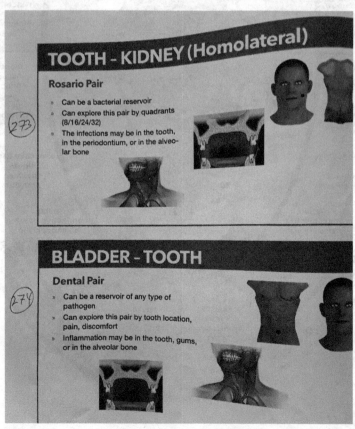

TOOTH - KIDNEY (Homolateral)

Rosario Pair

» Can be a bacterial reservoir
» Can explore this pair by quadrants (8/16/24/32)
» The infections may be in the tooth, in the periodontium, or in the alveolar bone

BLADDER - TOOTH

Dental Pair

» Can be a reservoir of any type of pathogen
» Can explore this pair by tooth location, pain, discomfort
» Inflammation may be in the tooth, gums, or in the alveolar bone

BiomagPet.Vet

To the right is images from a very large hematoma growth on my dog Oscar's testicle in Dec. 2019. In any other world of time I would of rushed him to an emergency veterinarian because he was in so much pain. I muscle scanned and found 3 pairs of placements for him as he lay in my lap with a towel over him while I administered the placements. He got outside of the house after the placements and I worried all night he was going to die.

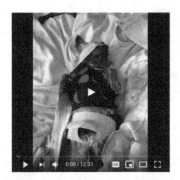

More Amazing Miracles Through Biomagetism & Dr. Magnetism Now Available for Healing What Ails You

The next morning, with great anticipation, he shows up with a big smile and tail wagging. As you can see from the image, the hematoma swelling had reduced greatly in size and the pain was nearly gone. Overnight! With only using magnets on him. Not only did I help heal my dog, Oscar, but saved a very large vet bill as well!

Magnetic therapy can also help to alleviate the pain in circumstances where arthritis and regular aging can limit their mobility. *Magnets for dogs and pets* will help improve blood circulation and will not interfere with any medication the pet might be already taking.

Scan your pet or animal the same way you would a human. Use the charts below to dial in specific placements and you can, and should, ask if there are any emotional issues associated with their issues and symtpoms. When Dr. Garcia scanned Oscar for me remotely, he told me that Oscar was lonely and wanted more time with me!

You may use a surrogate or I put a towel over the animal, if possible and apply the magnets to the towel draped over them. The same time frame applies as to how long to leave the magnets on.

Biomag Pet.Vet is still in its infancy. In fact, the vaccines given mandatorily to our pets is causing great harm, in some cases, to our beloved pets. Once a Veternairy Doctor learns BiomagHealing protocols, we will greatly advance our healing protocols for pets.

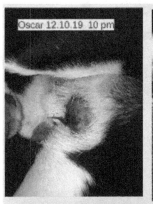

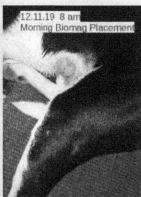

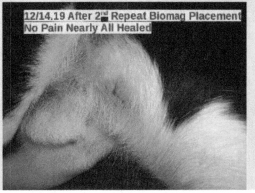

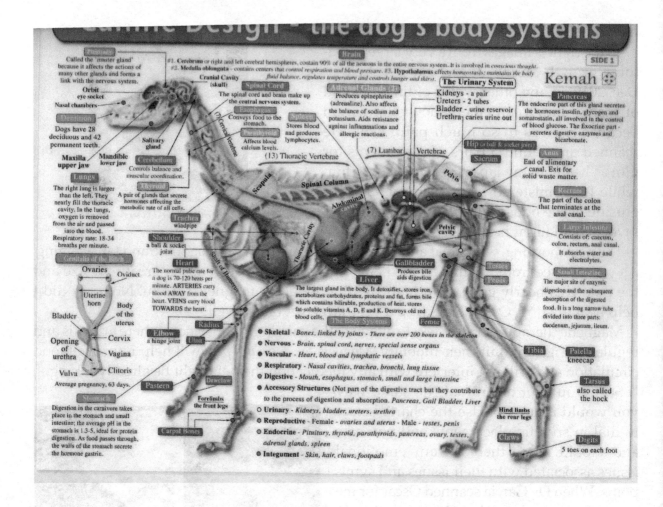

Canine Design - the dog's body systems

SIDE 1

Kemah

Pituitary
Called the 'master gland' because it affects the actions of many other glands and forms a link with the nervous system.

Orbit eye socket

Nasal chambers

Dentition
Dogs have 28 deciduous and 42 permanent teeth.

Maxilla upper jaw

Mandible lower jaw

Salivary gland

Cerebellum
Controls balance and muscular coordination.

Lungs
The right lung is larger than the left. They nearly fill the thoracic cavity. In the lungs, oxygen is removed from the air and passed into the blood. Respiratory rate: 18-34 breaths per minute.

Thyroid
A pair of glands that secrete hormones affecting the metabolic rate of all cells.

Trachea windpipe

Shoulder
a ball & socket joint

Genitalia of the Bitch
Ovaries
Oviduct
Uterine horn
Body of the uterus
Bladder
Cervix
Opening of urethra
Vagina
Vulva
Clitoris
Average pregnancy, 63 days.

Stomach
Digestion in the carnivore takes place in the stomach and small intestine; the average pH in the stomach is 1.3-5, ideal for protein digestion. As food passes through, the walls of the stomach secrete the hormone gastrin.

Heart
The normal pulse rate for a dog is 70-120 beats per minute. ARTERIES carry blood AWAY from the heart. VEINS carry blood TOWARDS the heart.

Elbow a hinge joint

Radius
Ulna

Pastern
Dewclaw
Forelimbs the front legs

Carpal Bones

Cranial Cavity (skull)

Spinal Cord
The spinal cord and brain make up the central nervous system.

Esophagus
Conveys food to the stomach.

Parathyroid
Affects blood calcium levels.

(7) Cervical Vertebrae

(13) Thoracic Vertebrae

Brain
#1. **Cerebrum** or right and left cerebral hemispheres, contain 90% of all the neurons in the entire nervous system. It is involved in *conscious thought*.
#2. **Medulla oblongata** - contains centers that *control respiration and blood pressure*. #3. **Hypothalamus** effects *homeostasis; maintains the body fluid balance, regulates temperature and controls hunger and thirst.*

Adrenal Glands (2)
Produces epinephrine (adrenaline). Also affects the balance of sodium and potassium. Aids resistance against inflammations and allergic reactions.

Spleen
Stores blood and produces lymphocytes.

(7) Lumbar   **Vertebrae**

Spinal Column

Scapula

Spinal Column

Abdominal Cavity

Thoracic Cavity

Shaft of Humerus

Liver
The largest gland in the body. It detoxifies, stores iron, metabolizes carbohydrates, proteins and fat, forms bile which contains bilirubin, production of heat, stores fat-soluble vitamins A, D, E and K. Destroys old red blood cells.

Gallbladder
Produces bile aids digestion

The Urinary System
Kidneys - a pair
Ureters - 2 tubes
Bladder - urine reservoir
Urethra caries urine out

Pancreas
The endocrine part of this gland secretes the hormones insulin, glycogen and somatostatin, all involved in the control of blood glucose. The Exocrine part secretes digestive enzymes and bicarbonate.

Hip (or ball & socket joint)
Sacrum

Pelvis

Pelvic cavity

Anus
End of alimentary canal. Exit for solid waste matter.

Rectum
The part of the colon that terminates at the anal canal.

Large Intestine
Consists of: caecum, colon, rectum, anal canal. It absorbs water and electrolytes.

Small Intestine
The major site of enzymic digestion and the subsequent absorption of the digested food. It is a long narrow tube divided into three parts: duodenum, jejunum, ileum.

Testes
Penis

Femur

The Body Systems
- **Skeletal** - *Bones, linked by joints - There are over 200 bones in the skeleton*
- **Nervous** - *Brain, spinal cord, nerves, special sense organs*
- **Vascular** - *Heart, blood and lymphatic vessels*
- **Respiratory** - *Nasal cavities, trachea, bronchi, lung tissue*
- **Digestive** - *Mouth, esophagus, stomach, small and large intestine*
- **Accessory Structures** (*Not part of the digestive tract but they contribute to the process of digestion and absorption. Pancreas, Gall Bladder, Liver*
- **Urinary** - *Kidneys, bladder, ureters, urethra*
- **Reproductive** - *Female - ovaries and uterus - Male - testes, penis*
- **Endocrine** - *Pituitary, thyroid, parathyroids, pancreas, ovary, testes, adrenal glands, spleen*
- **Integument** - *Skin, hair, claws, footpads*

Tibia
Patella kneecap

Tarsus also called the hock

Hind limbs the rear legs

Claws

Digits
5 toes on each foot

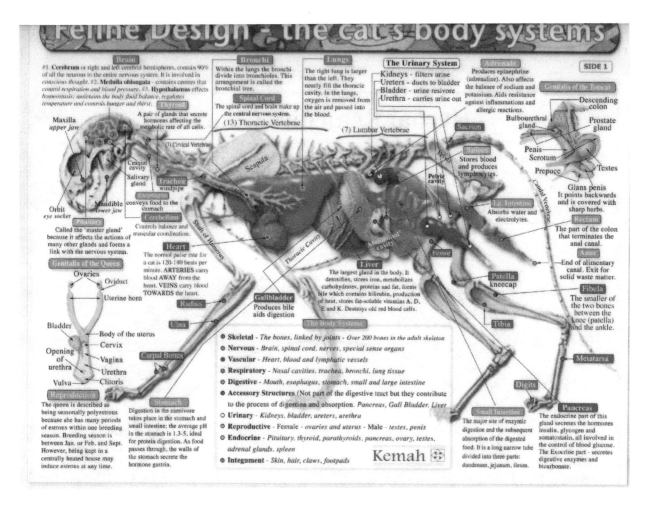

Feline Design - the cat's body systems

SIDE 1

Brain
#1. **Cerebrum** or right and left cerebral hemispheres, contain 90% of all the neurons in the entire nervous system. It is involved in *conscious thought*. #2. **Medulla oblongata** - contains centres that *control respiration and blood pressure*. #3. **Hypothalamus** effects *homeostasis; maintains the body fluid balance, regulates temperature and controls hunger and thirst*.

Thyroid
A pair of glands that secrete hormones affecting the metabolic rate of all cells.

Spinal Cord
The spinal cord and brain make up the central nervous system.

Bronchi
Within the lungs the bronchi divide into bronchioles. This arrangement is called the bronchial tree.

Lungs
The right lung is larger than the left. They nearly fill the thoracic cavity. In the lungs, oxygen is removed from the air and passed into the blood.

The Urinary System
Kidneys - filters urine
Ureters - ducts to bladder
Bladder - urine resivore
Urethra - carries urine out

Adrenals
Produces epinephrine (adrenaline). Also affects the balance of sodium and potassium. Aids resistance against inflammations and allergic reactions.

Genitalia of the Tomcat
Descending colon
Bulbourethral gland
Prostate gland
Penis
Scrotum
Prepuce
Testes
Glans penis
It points backwards and is covered with sharp barbs.

Pituitary
Called the 'master gland' because it affects the actions of many other glands and forms a link with the nervous system.

Cerebellum
Controls balance and muscular coordination.

Esophagus
conveys food to the stomach

Trachea
windpipe

Salivary gland

Cranial cavity

Mandible *lower jaw*

Maxilla *upper jaw*

Orbit *eye socket*

Heart
The normal pulse rate for a cat is 120-180 beats per minute. ARTERIES carry blood AWAY from the heart. VEINS carry blood TOWARDS the heart.

Liver
The largest gland in the body. It detoxifies, stores iron, metabolizes carbohydrates, proteins and fat, forms bile which contains bilirubin, production of heat, stores fat-soluble vitamins A, D, E and K. Destroys old red blood cells.

Spleen
Stores blood and produces lymphocytes.

Lg. Intestine
Absorbs water and electrolytes.

Rectum
The part of the colon that terminates the anal canal.

Anus
End of alimentary canal. Exit for solid waste matter.

Fibula
The smaller of the two bones between the knee (patella) and the ankle.

Patella
kneecap

Genitalia of the Queen
Ovaries
Oviduct
Uterine horn
Bladder
Body of the uterus
Cervix
Opening of urethra
Vagina
Urethra
Vulva
Clitoris

Radius
Ulna
Carpal Bones

Gallbladder
Produces bile aids digestion

Tibia
Metatarsa
Digits

Reproduction
The queen is described as being seasonally polyestrous because she has many periods of estrous within one breeding season. Breeding season is between Jan. or Feb. and Sept. However, being kept in a centrally heated house may induce estrous at any time.

Stomach
Digestion in the carnivore takes place in the stomach and small intestine; the average pH in the stomach is 1.3-5, ideal for protein digestion. As food passes through, the walls of the stomach secrete the hormone gastrin.

The Body Systems
● **Skeletal** - *The bones, linked by joints · Over 200 bones in the adult skeleton*
● **Nervous** - *Brain, spinal cord, nerves, special sense organs*
● **Vascular** - *Heart, blood and lymphatic vessels*
● **Respiratory** - *Nasal cavities, trachea, bronchi, lung tissue*
● **Digestive** - *Mouth, esophagus, stomach, small and large intestine*
● **Accessory Structures** (Not part of the digestive tract but they contribute to the process of digestion and absorption. *Pancreas, Gall Bladder, Liver*
○ **Urinary** - *Kidneys, bladder, ureters, urethra*
● **Reproductive** - *Female - ovaries and uterus · Male - testes, penis*
● **Endocrine** - *Pituitary, thyroid, parathyroids, pancreas, ovary, testes, adrenal glands, spleen*
● **Integument** - *Skin, hair, claws, footpads*

Kemah

Small Intestine
The major site of enzymic digestion and the subsequent absorption of the digested food. It is a long narrow tube divided into three parts: duodenum, jejunum, ileum.

Pancreas
The endocrine part of this gland secretes the hormones insulin, glycogen and somatostatin, all involved in the control of blood glucose. The Exocrine part - secretes digestive enzymes and bicarbonate.

(7) Cervical Vertebrae
(13) Thoracic Vertebrae
(7) Lumbar Vertebrae
Scapula
Sacrum
Shaft of Humerus
Thoracic Cavity
Abdominal cavity
Pelvic cavity
Kidney
Femur
Caudal Vertebrae

Use these charts to muscle test your souls after session work to suggest healing remedies and supplements.

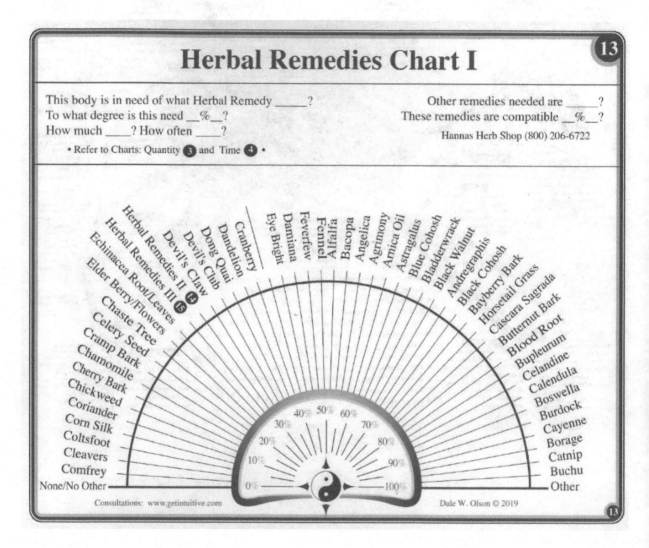

Herbal Remedies Chart I

This body is in need of what Herbal Remedy _____?
To what degree is this need __%__?
How much ____? How often ____?
• Refer to Charts: Quantity ③ and Time ④ •

Other remedies needed are _____?
These remedies are compatible __%__?

Hannas Herb Shop (800) 206-6722

Herbal Remedies III ⑮
Herbal Remedies II
Herbal Remedies I
Echinacea Root/Leaves
Elder Berry/Flowers
Chaste Tree
Celery Seed
Cramp Bark
Chamomile
Cherry Bark
Chickweed
Coriander
Corn Silk
Coltsfoot
Cleavers
Comfrey
None/No Other

Devil's Claw ⑭
Devil's Club
Dong Quai
Dandelion
Cranberry
Eye Bright
Damiana
Feverfew
Fennel
Alfalfa
Bacopa
Angelica
Agrimony
Arnica Oil
Astragalus
Blue Cohosh
Bladderwrack
Black Walnut
Andregraphis
Black Cohosh
Bayberry Bark
Horsetail Grass
Cascara Sagrada
Butternut Bark
Blood Root
Bupleurum
Celandine
Calendula
Boswella
Burdock
Cayenne
Borage
Catnip
Buchu
Other

40% 50% 60%
30% 70%
20% 80%
10% 90%
0% 100%

Consultations: www.getintuitive.com

Dale W. Olson © 2019

Herbal Remedies Chart II

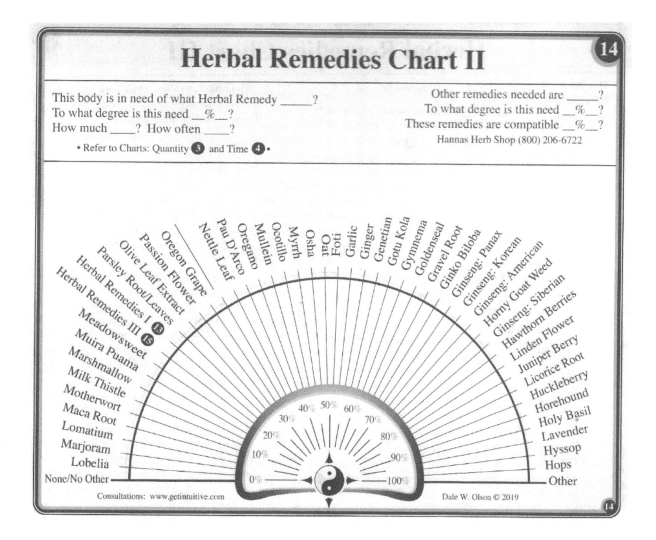

This body is in need of what Herbal Remedy _____?
To what degree is this need __%__?
How much ____? How often ____?

• Refer to Charts: Quantity ❸ and Time ❹ •

Other remedies needed are _____?
To what degree is this need __%__?
These remedies are compatible __%__?

Hannas Herb Shop (800) 206-6722

Consultations: www.getintuitive.com

Dale W. Olson © 2019

Herbal Remedies Chart III

15

This body is in need of what Herbal Remedy _____?
To what degree is this need __%__?
How much _____? How often _____?

  • Refer to Charts: Quantity **3** and Time **4** •

Other remedies needed are _____?
To what degree is this need __%__?
These remedies are compatible __%__?

Hannas Herb Shop (800) 206-6722

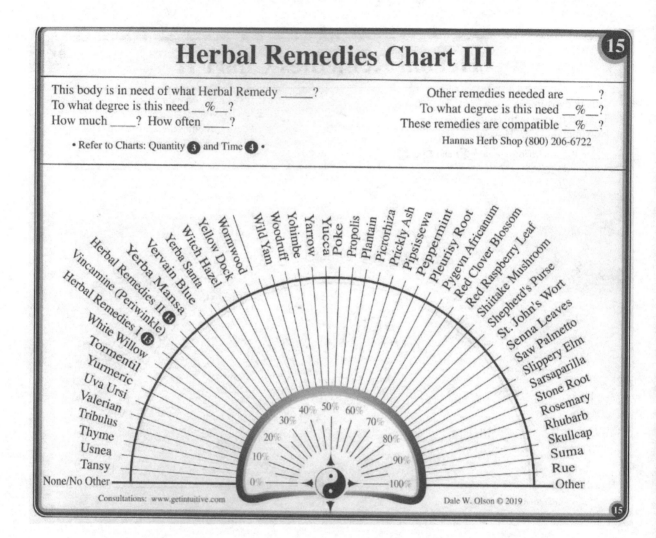

Consultations: www.getintuitive.com

Dale W. Olson © 2019

15

Vitamin Chart

5

This body is in need of _____ vitamin(s)?
To what degree is this need __%__?
How much ____? How often ____?
   • Refer to Charts: Quantity ❸ and Time ❹ •

This body needs _____ vitamin(s) to
    be increased by __%__?
This body is in excess of_____ vitamin?
    To what degree __%__?

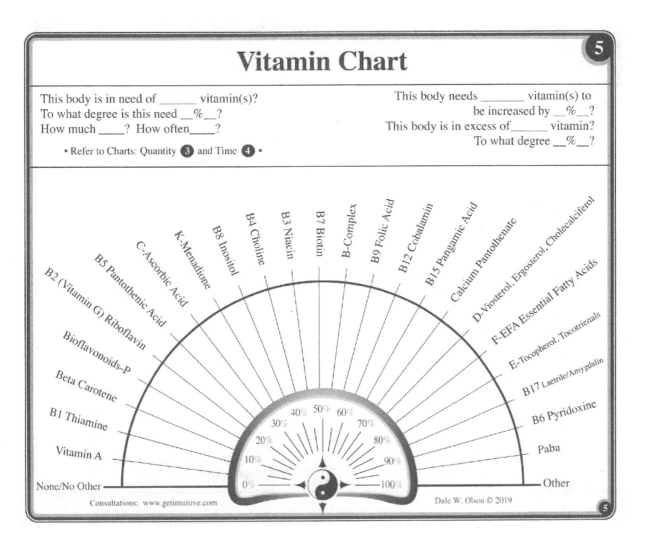

Consultations: www.getintuitive.com   Dale W. Olson © 2019

Essential Oils Chart

12

This body is in need of what Essential Oil(s) _____?

To what degree is this need ___?___?

How much ___? How Often___?

    • Refer to Charts: Quantity **3** and Time **4** •

What other Essential Oils are needed _____?

To what degree are these oils compatibile ___%___?

    • For Essential Oils see www.getintuitive.com

or contact Young Living Essential Oils •

• See Volume II for expanded Essential

Oils list + Blended Oils Chart •

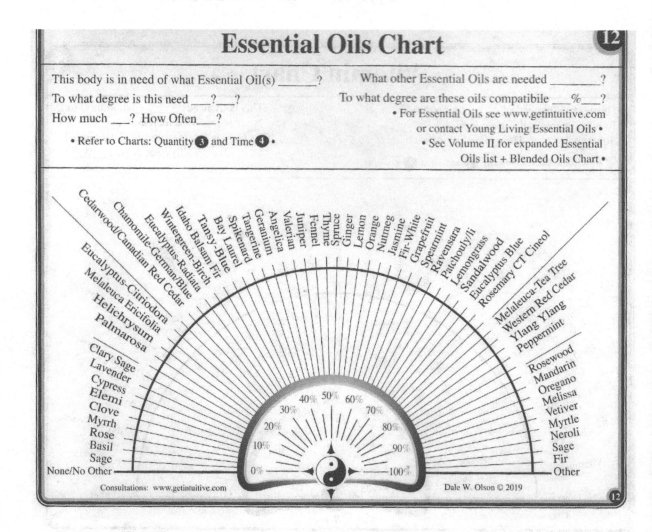

Consultations: www.getintuitive.com

Dale W. Olson © 2019

12

Essential & Trace Minerals Chart

This body is in need of what mineral(s)_____?
This body is in need of what trace mineral(s)_____?
To what degree is this need ___%___?
How much___? How often ___?
   • Refer to Charts: Quantity ❸ and Time ❹ •

This body has an excess of what mineral _____?
To what degree __%__?
How much___? How often ___?

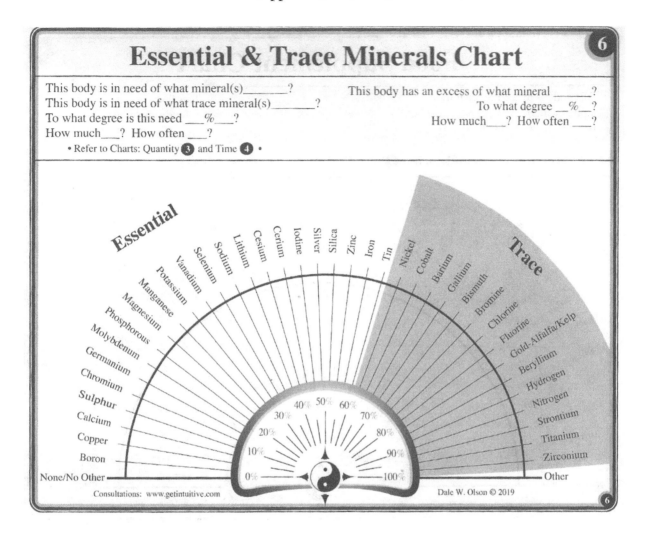

Consultations: www.getintuitive.com

Dale W. Olson © 2019

Food Supplement Chart

9

This body is in need of what food supplement(s) _____? To what degree is this need __%__? How much _____, how often _____?

• Refer to Charts: Quantity **3** and Time **4** •

This body is in excess of what food supplement(s) _____? To what degree __%__?

• See Volume II for the expanded version •

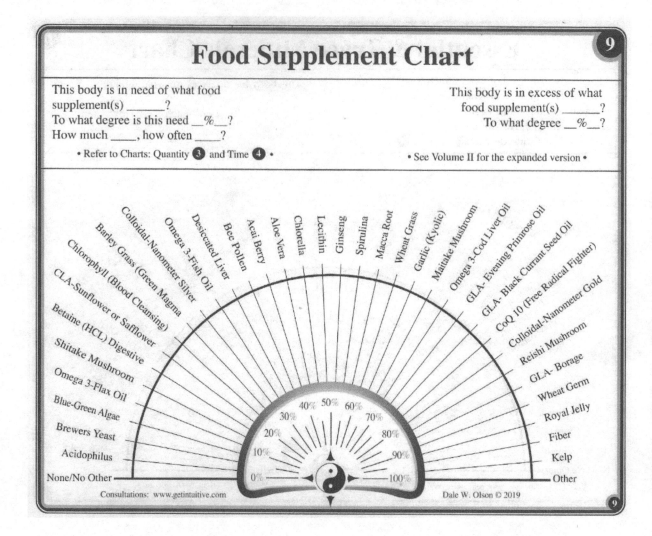

Consultations: www.getintuitive.com

Dale W. Olson © 2019

9

Appendix III

Testimonials

D r. Garcia tells the story in his 5-day intensive workshop about how his wife's father fell down the stairs at his home one day and cracked his head wide open hitting the freezer door edge as he fell.

The gash was so deep the bone could be seen. While the family was calling for emergency assistance to take his wife's father to the emergency room, Dr. Garcia had the presence of mind to muscle test to see if he could assist his father-in-law solely with magnets, pearle crème and steri-strips to help close the wound.

As you can clearly see from the images below, the father-in-law experienced no pain, significantly reduced swelling and with 3 months no scarring. Never having to the emergency room, see doctors or take any pills, saving him thousands of dollars in medical bills. EVERYONE NEEDS TO LEARN THIS FIRST AID HEALING PROTOCOL.

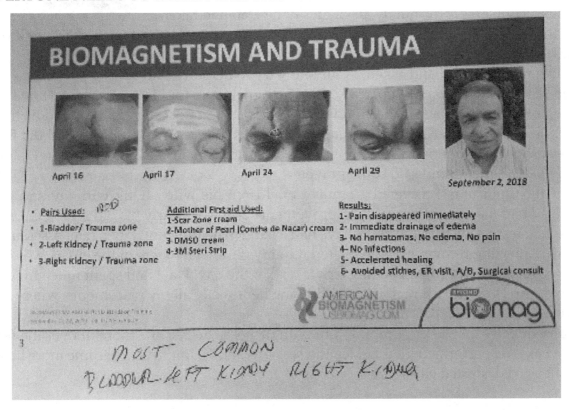

Sometimes the soul still has to go through their issues to learn what they came here to learn and the Universe is telling you they are not ready yet for you to do placements to help them.

My recent example was my 94-year young father who they discovered a lump on his neck and got a biopsy that came back as a cancer phenomenon. I offered my BiomagHealing services but was dismissed outright by my medical family...what did I know and who am I to think I could put magnets on a surrogate and help my dad?... I'm sure they all just dismissed me outright. I muscle tested and asked "can I help Dad now?" and got a firm, "No" which was very disheartening.

Growing up in a medical family (doctors, dentist, nurse, HMO, etc.), they were all discussing what route to take whether they should administer Chemotherapy, Surgery, Immunotherapy, etc and after great discussion decided on the Immunotherapy route that was very dangerous for someone my Dad's age. The National Institute of Health had even said it was "untested adequately on seniors" and that there "appeared to be a higher than normal mortality rate when used by seniors". I sent the info to the medical family and they still went ahead.

Just 5 days after he received immunotherapy, his wife, a 30 yr. registered nurse, sent the family an email saying Dad had taken a turn for the worst, could hardly get up, no appetite, and had brain fog. She did not know if he had much longer, he could not walk, was very cold and had little energy.

I then muscle tested and asked, "Can I now try to help my Dad NOW???" The answer came back "yes". That night I placed over 45 magnet pairs for him on my surrogate I use for remote healing. I had no idea if it would work as I did not see my father and he lived a couple of hours away, but my scanning, using Dr. Garcia's protocols, located the false tumor as well as placements for temperature regulation, balance, fatigue and viral issues. I did the placements and said some prayers.

The next morning, I received a family email from his wife saying with joy and glee that Dad had made a "remarkable improvement" and was nearly his old self again! This brought me great joy to know I may have had a hand in helping my father. (Her assessment as to his amazing recovery, as she related it to my family members in the email, was that his recovery was due to him getting a new walker the day! Ha! I had spent much time on my workup I sent her the night before showing her exactly all my placements, where and why, yet it was the walker that did it!!)

Subsequently they kept pumping him with drugs as he became more ill over the next few weeks so I performed BiomagHealing sessions and he improved, became more lucid, wasn't as cold, started eating, etc.

Then they administered more drugs as his lump in his throat, the original issue became very inflamed and other cysts developed. Muscle testing told me the drugs were causing the issues. As he slipped further and further, my well intentional medical family pumped him with morphine and more drugs.

Two months later, my father passed in his sleep. Did the immune therapy drugs accelerate his passing? Or was it the vaccines?? My muscle testing told me "yes on both"!

We need BiomagHospice protocols urgently. I saw firsthand how BiomagHealing can make an elderly's transition much more comfortable without morphine and all the other drugs that they give them.

Jen Colombo -Connecticut

I feel AMAZING and full of life. The weight of all the emotional burden I was carrying for the last month or so has been lifted. I feel it it my face, my eyes feel larger and I am aware of the constant upward smile of my mouth. My cells feel like they are dancing & vibrating the way I love them to be, happy. I was able to finally meditate deeply again after weeks of struggle. I also feel like my energy field has expanded out so far and I am able to move energy on myself again the way I could months ago. And it's not going unnoticed by those close as well as clients. My husband commented to me the following day how since the day prior my whole attitude & demeanor completely shifted. I feel positive and hopeful again.The session set me back on the course I know I am supposed to be on that I had veered from. And it feels incredible to be back on track to working towards being a glowing light. Many, many thanks Dr. Garcia.

Marsha Nolan –New Jersey

Hi Dr. Garcia, As a recap, some of the major problems that I have had started back around 1990 were multiple chemical sensitivity, chronic fatigue, fibromyalgia, colitis and Hashimoto's thyroiditis. I never went to a mall because of all the chemical and perfume smells and I could not even stand cooking smells. In 2004 I was diagnosed with Primary Sclerosing Cholangitis (PSC) a degenerative liver disease.

Two and a half years ago when my primary doctor at Stockton Family Practice recommended I try Biomagnetism therapy using magnets. I really thought he had flipped and I wanted to reject this until I spoke with you. We resonated almost immediately since you used words that were similar to things I believed in, they were similar to other holistic natural treatments I had tried in the past, so I gave myself the opportunity to try yet another system. I had been in pain for over 20 years starting from a tailbone break onward, after the first treatment all this pain went away for 4 weeks. The treatment plan was supposed to be once a month for several months until I could gradually extend my sessions. Today, I have been able to extend this time period for up to 5 months! This is Ok with me because if and when I return to any discomfort or other problems I know what

I can do and where I can go! I do live in reality, I know I must adhere to my GF diet, no dairy and muscle test foods always. You have balanced my organs to the point where they are functioning much better and to think about it, I have not had any digestive problems lately. I now understand that our bodies are complex systems that can heal themselves when given the proper pH and magnetic.

On another note, I would love to share my latest colonoscopy test results. It has been 3 years since my last colonoscopy test and at that time I still had colitis. There is very definite evidence that I had very active Colitis in the past due to the extensive scarring still present in the films. This scarring does not cause any problems. At this time I have NO COLITIS AT ALL, NO POLYPS OR ANY PRE CANCER CELLS. I do a lot of other internal exercises to stay healthy, but your Biomagnetism therapy is the only really different thing that I have done for the last 2 and 1/2 years of the 3 since my last test. Additionally, test results for the PSC have been consistently normal with no elevation at all. No matter what other system I may try I will always remain a patient of Biomagnetism therapy, for semiannual tweaking or whenever necessary. It can be easy through stress to get unbalanced and I know now where to go if that happens again.

I have never believed the old adage that "old age meant you had to have aches and pains" but when I was faced with the above named diseases it was a challenge to keep the faith and not fall into the trap of believing what they say. I am a pretty strong willed person so I tried many different modalities to regain my health. I believe that lots of things out there do work but not for everyone. What I can say is that Biomagnetism therapy is the only therapy that has made a significant difference in my life. I have more energy now than when I was much younger, and my aches and pains and degenerative conditions have reversed themselves.

I now understand that we CAN regain our health even after the retirement years! You just need to find the right path!

Jairo Q. – New Jersey Fibromyalgia, Allergies, Chronic back pain

After 10 years of illness, I was referred to Dr. Garcia by my medical doctor who, like dozens before him, couldn't relieve my symptoms. Suffering from severe gastrointestinal issues, parasites, fungal infections, viruses, lyme disease and co-infections, adrenal fatigue, PVCs, profound fatigue, hypothyroidism, ovarian cysts, muscle and joint pain–the list is too long for this page–I thought there would be no end. After the first biomagnetism therapy, my body started to feel calm instead of in a state of panic, and less like it was being eaten from the inside out from all the infections that I had raging inside of me. Aches and pains improved, vision and skin integrity, and diarrhea better controlled, along with some unexpected improvements such as a fungal rash disappearing within 3 days after having it for over 10 years, and bleeding and cracked lips healed. We have learned so much from him such as how much I was specifically affected by EMF and radiation, heavy metals, food allergens, mold, and how to do our best to prevent illness in the first place.

I have learned and experienced personally with Dr. Garcia's sessions how the cause of so many illnesses, from a headache to cancer, can be caused by pathogens. As a physical therapist with a doctoral degree, I am blown away at how quickly chronic muscle and joint pain, neurological symptoms, as well as leg length discrepancy can be impacted sometimes instantly with this approach! Biomagnetism addresses the underlying causes of so many symptoms.

It has been a long journey for me, since I have been sick for so many years. I will continue to improve with biomagnetism and am very blessed that my medical doctor and Dr. Garcia can work as a team with prescriptions, supplements, etc. Most of all, I have hope knowing that I have seen improvement after so many years of failed medical treatments, and that I will continue to get healthier.

Sara B. – Pennsylvania Lyme disease, Adrenal fatigue

Dr. Garcia has been a blessing not only to me but to my entire family; I first came to know of the wonders of biogmagnetism when Dr. Garcia treated my mom, who used to suffer from fibromyalgia, after a couple of therapies her recovery was amazing and she is now enjoying a healthy life. After seeing the results the therapy had on my mother's health I decided to give it a try myself. I have suffered from severe allergies since I was about 16 years old; I had already been through a series of medical treatments that only relieved my allergies temporarily. After the first biomagnetism therapy, my allergy symptoms started to decrease considerably, to the point where I didn't have to take my daily allergy medication. I encouraged my wife to receive several therapies as she had chronic back pain and we had also been trying to get pregnant. After a couple of therapies, my wife's back pain decreased considerably and a couple of months later we found out we were pregnant! We were blessed with a healthy girl who is also enjoying the benefits of biomagnetism.

Teeth Issues

Hi Jamie. I'm away in Costa Rica at an ayahuasca retreat. I wanted to let you know that my tooth pain is still gone! The placement of black on my root canal tooth and red on my kidney seems to have helped immediately.

I had literally gone to the dentist before our session and had an x-ray and they said that I needed a root canal because the nerve was very inflamed. I really didn't want a root canal and was planning to have the tooth pulled, so far, two weeks later, it's still feeling fine. ~ **Talysia Allen**

Setting Up Your Business as a Biomag Healer

The BiomagHealing Business model is wide open for you to create whatever healing business you wish to persue and create.

I have a Biomag store selling my services of session work, individual consultations, workshops on applied biomagnetism as well as sell magnetic waters sleeves, magnets and bed toppers.

DO NOT be afraid to charge money for your services. You are saving them possibly thousands and thousands of dollars in medical bills and prescriptions and factor in all the time you have spent learning and practicing and not getting paid. I offer a sliding scale since I feel this healing protocol should be available to all.

Make sure to keep records of your session work and cover yourself by this disclosure before beginning session work.

Qualifier Statement

"Certified Biomagnetic Practioners, unless separately licensed to do so, do not diagnose or prescribe for medical or psychological conditions nor claim to prevent, treat, mitigate or cure such conditions, nor provide diagnosis, care, treatment or rehabilitation of individuals, nor apply medical, mental health or human development principles, but rather provide traditional ministerial counseling, bioenergetic, biofeedback, herbal and/or nutritional modalities that may offer therapeutic benefit by supporting normal structure and function."

Here is a legalese words list of what words you can use and what ones may get the Medical Mafia after you. I also highly suggest Corbet Reports excellent takedown of how and why Western Medicine was created and its purpose. https://ipfs.io/ipns/QmNqHuSVuufkB-KK1LHtoUmKETobZriC1o5uoiXSoLX2i3K/episode-286-rockefeller-medicine/

Banned Words	Safe Words
Client/Patient	Soul
Facilitator	Doctor
Treatment	Protocol
Diagnose	Scan
Prevent	Strenghten
Prescribe	Suggest
Prevent	Reduce/Modify

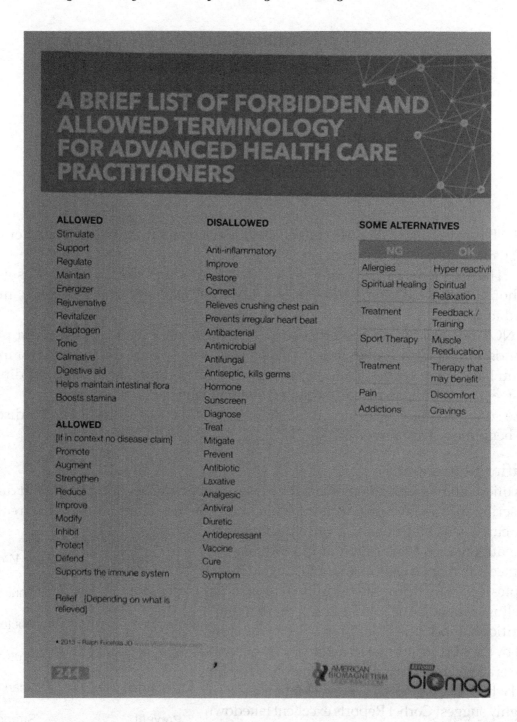

A BRIEF LIST OF FORBIDDEN AND ALLOWED TERMINOLOGY FOR ADVANCED HEALTH CARE PRACTITIONERS

ALLOWED
Stimulate
Support
Regulate
Maintain
Energizer
Rejuvenative
Revitalizer
Adaptogen
Tonic
Calmative
Digestive aid
Helps maintain intestinal flora
Boosts stamina

ALLOWED
[If in context no disease claim]
Promote
Augment
Strengthen
Reduce
Improve
Modify
Inhibit
Protect
Defend
Supports the immune system

Relief   [Depending on what is relieved]

* 2013 – Ralph Fucetola JD

DISALLOWED
Anti-inflammatory
Improve
Restore
Correct
Relieves crushing chest pain
Prevents irregular heart beat
Antibacterial
Antimicrobial
Antifungal
Antiseptic, kills germs
Hormone
Sunscreen
Diagnose
Treat
Mitigate
Prevent
Antibiotic
Laxative
Analgesic
Antiviral
Diuretic
Antidepressant
Vaccine
Cure
Symptom

SOME ALTERNATIVES

NG	OK
Allergies	Hyper reactivity
Spiritual Healing	Spiritual Relaxation
Treatment	Feedback / Training
Sport Therapy	Muscle Reeducation
Treatment	Therapy that may benefit
Pain	Discomfort
Addictions	Cravings

AMERICAN BIOMAGNETISM

biomag

Appendix V

BiomagHealer Goods and Services

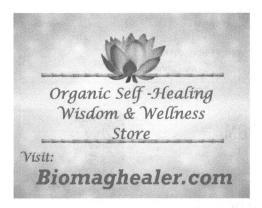
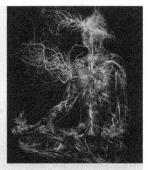

ULTRACREME, 50ML

$95.00

Natural skin nourishment for skin beautification support, for external application for health support, and cosmetic enhancement.

The best and longest lasting results are seen with skin that is most damaged or neglected. Restores youthful and healthy tone and texture.

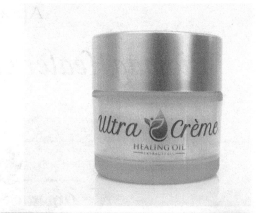

SCIATICREME, 59GM

$95.00

RAPID RELIEF OF SCIATICA SYMPTOMS OF PAIN, NEUROPATHY AND NUMBNESS AND, IN MOST CASES, EXTREMITY WEAKNESS.

The new technology of the Theraben process unleashes the power of homeopathy in a new and powerful way. This proprietary formulation gives Theraben the power to do what a universal pain remedy should do, without the adverse effects*, and, in most cases, it succeeds with flying colors.

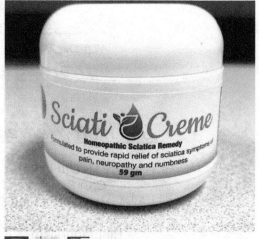

MYCO-3, 10ML

$49.00

A proprietary blend used to support treatments of mold problems.

Recommended Usage: Use MYCO-3 in conjunction with Calm Balm or TheraCreme.

Application: Consult with your healthcare provider and use as directed. (see below note)

Do not use if allergic to any ingredients.

Ingredients: Coconut Oil, Oregano Oil, Grapefruit Seed Oil*, Grape Seed Oil*, and Castor Oil*. *Proprietary Theraben® process.

Note: Consult with your physician. Do not do this protocol on your own. Only work with a physician familiar with using this protocol.

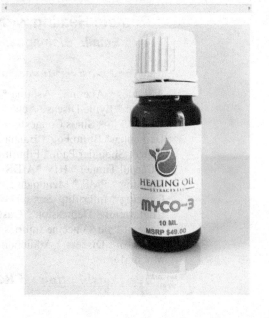

N52 RARE EARTH NEODYMIUM MAGNETS

$15.00

15.00 **per Pair**

Minimum Gauss Strength: 1100.

Magnets for Biomagnetic Healing are encased in a vinyl sleeve covering to provide ease of use and longevity. Black color is for negative and Red color is for positive magnetic polarities. Magnets generate several fields of energy.

Magnets for use in Biomagnetism must have at least 1,000 surfaces Gauss so that they may provide the proper benefit. The magnets are sold in pairs only. They are encased in a water-resistant synthetic leather material so that they can be washed and should not wear out for years.

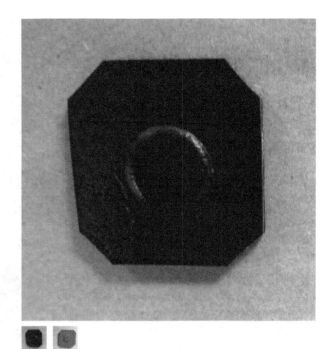

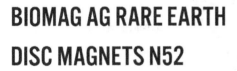

BIOMAG AG RARE EARTH DISC MAGNETS N52

$32.00

Size: 5/8 x 1/4 Inch, 10-Pack

Magnetism is Earth's Natural Remedy

Use BiomagAg magnets to enrich and build stronger plants, spur faster growth from seedlings to fruition and can generate greater yields of crops and produce.

The Earth has a magnetic core. She is also rich in magnetite. Adding magnets to plants and soil greatly enhances the life energy forces to enhance plant growth. You can place magnets around your seeds when you sow them. Add them to your gardens and bury them in your soil to create a magnetized growing environment.

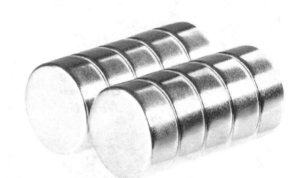

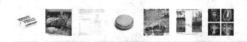

MAGNETIC VORTEX STRUCTURED WATER SLEEVE

$50.00

The item has 4 paired magnets inside the sleeve. The magnetic energy will create structured water from where you put the sleeve. You can put it on your sink faucet (see image); where the water comes into your home or garden; at the hose bib; under the sink (but you may need two: (one for hot pipe, one for cold), or on the shower head, bath tube nozzle, etc.

Installation Instructions

You can install the sleeve with two zip ties or tape with gorilla tape or duct tape. Make sure to follow the arrows where the water enters the sleeve to exit in the direction of flow INTO your house.

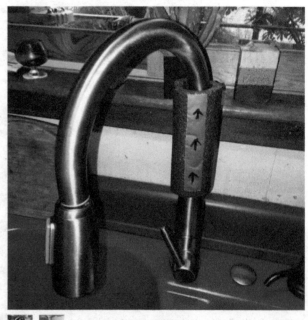

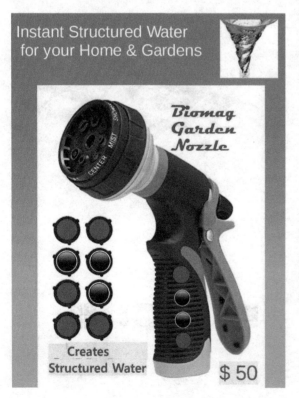

Instant Structured Water for your Home & Gardens

Biomag Garden Nozzle

Creates Structured Water

$ 50

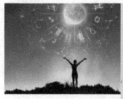

ASTROLOGY READINGS.

Do you know what your life purpose is and plans for you incarnating to this world at this time? Would you like to better understand what assets and roadblocks are in your natal chart? Would you like to better understand your energetic strengths and weaknesses so you can cope with life more easily? Sessions are with Jamie Lee.

$125 /One-Hour Natal Chart Reading via Zoom or phone call

Schedule

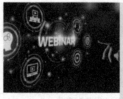

EDUCATIONAL WEBINARS.

Biomagnetism Healing Experiences and Effect, Session I & Session II [4-hour webinar]

Dr. Luis Garcia is one of the most advanced Biomagnetic Practioners in the world today. He has been applying Biomagnetic Healing for the past 13 years. In each of these 2-hour presentations you will learn from the master himself about the effects of Biomag Healing and how to heal yourself with magnets.

Session I & II: $50 with Dr. Luis Garcia

Schedule

Bibliography

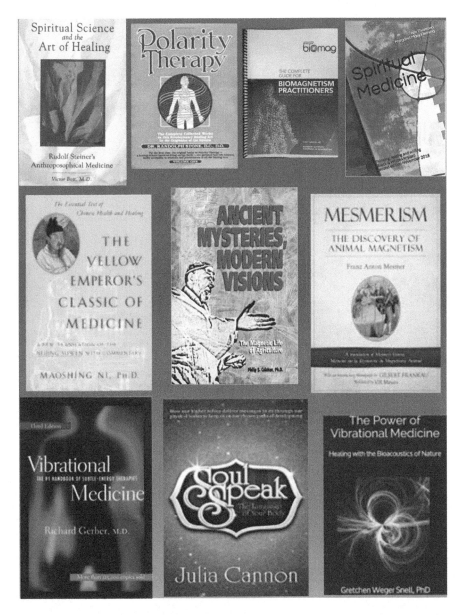

The Magnetic Effect Magnetism   Albert Roy Davis
Paramagnetism   Philip s. Callahan Ph.D
Healing with Magnets   Gary Null Ph.D
Archangel Raphael   Doreen Virture

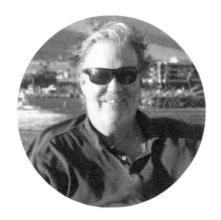

Hi,

I am autodidactic, meaning 'self-taught'. I did not do well being schooled but learned to think and learn for myself by reading, thinking and experiencing life.

I was formerly an Institutional Sales Trading Analysts on Wall Street beginning in 1985 before opening up my own JWL Investment Banking Inc. company in 1992. Previously. I worked as a mortgage loan officer for residential sales.

I received a B.S. in Business Marketing from San Diego State University in 1980 and returned to school in 2006 to get my GreenMba degree from New College in Santa Rosa, California.

Activism: Biomagnetic Healer. Biodynamic Community Farmer. Author/Writer/Blogger. Deep State Researcher. Ollie Foundation (Charity). Mr. Glean. Measure S. Image for Success. Alternative Healer. Food Runners. Freegive.me. Unvaxxed,

Hobbies: Community building. Farming. Reading. Learning. Yoga. Dot Connecting. Meditating.

Talents: Independent Thinker. Astrology readings. Revisionist Historian. Educator to the Educators. Run Real Life 'Future Essential Skills Camps' on Permaculture for youth during summer months at our ranch.

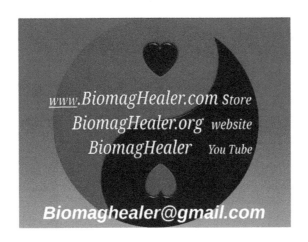

Dr. Magnetism's Social Media

BiomagHealer
https://www.biomaghealer.com/
https://www.youtube.com/channel/UCOslwW_HoMORuSFCj6Hk8_g
Facebook: BiomagHealer
Discord: BiomagHealer

Biomag Healing Store
https://biomaghealer.org/

You Tube
Aplanetruth11 https://www.youtube.com/channel/UCgc7T3SbIfEw9HTliB7WhuA
Aplanetruth10 https://www.youtube.com/channel/UCuVGYuVkQH6-EeRavJhY9ig
Aplanetruth9 https://www.youtube.com/channel/UCkbTwxFt8szbwwJj0pKQVAg
Aplanetruth8 https://www.youtube.com/channel/UCK4zVdKp4Ev2nZj_B3jxyLw
Aplanetruth3 https://www.youtube.com/channel/UCbM5aiq-du38a05SfseMTPg
Aplanetruth12 https://www.youtube.com/channel/UCyC1htf4qm9h4AR-5MX_LRA

Websites
Aplanetruth.info   https://aplanetruth.info/
Tabublog.com   https://tabublog.com/

Vaxxine
avvi.info

My Books Free on .pdf

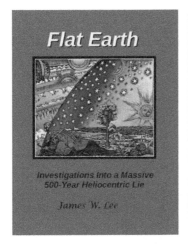
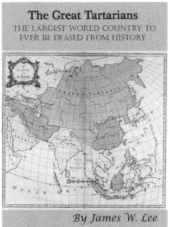

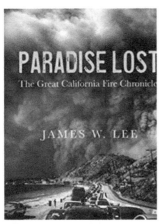
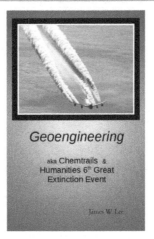

One World Tartarianshttps://aplanetruth.info/2020/09/28/one-world-tartarian-book-launch-incl-free-pdf/

Geoengineering aka Chemtrails
https://aplanetruth.info/2020/01/12/free-book-geongineering-aka-chemtrails/

Paradise Lost: The Great California Fires Chronicles
https://planetruthblog.files.wordpress.com/2020/08/ccthe-california-fire-chronicles-first-edition.pdf

Flat Earth; Investigations Into a 500 Yr. Massive Life
https://planetruthblog.files.wordpress.com/2020/08/fe-color-final-book-7-24-173.pdf

Made in the USA
Monee, IL
19 March 2025

14233859R20142